Critical Care of Patients with Mental Health Issues

Guest Editor

SUSAN MACE WEEKS, DNP, RN, CNS, LMFT, FAAN

CRITICAL CARE NURSING CLINICS OF NORTH AMERICA

www.ccnursing.theclinics.com

Consulting Editor
JANET FOSTER, PhD, RN, CNS

March 2012 • Volume 24 • Number 1

SAUNDERS an imprint of ELSEVIER, Inc.

W.B. SAUNDERS COMPANY
A Division of Elsevier Inc.

Elsevier Inc., 1600 John F. Kennedy Blvd., Suite 1800, Philadelphia, PA 19103-2899

http://www.theclinics.com

CRITICAL CARE NURSING CLINICS OF NORTH AMERICA Volume 24, Number 1
March 2012 ISSN 0899-5885, ISBN-13: 978-1-4557-4451-0

Editor: Katie Hartner
Developmental Editor: Donald E. Mumford

Critical Care Nursing Clinics of North America (ISSN 0899-5885) is published quarterly by Elsevier Inc., 360 Park Avenue South, New York, NY 10010-1710. Months of issue are March, June, September, and December. Business and Editorial Offices: 1600 John F. Kennedy Blvd., Suite 1800, Philadelphia, PA 19103-2899. Periodicals postage paid at New York, NY and additional mailing offices. Subscription prices are $144.00 per year for US individuals, $296.00 per year for US institutions, $76.00 per year for US students and residents, $192.00 per year for Canadian individuals, $371.00 per year for Canadian institutions, $219.00 per year for international individuals, $371.00 per year for international institutions and $111.00 per year for Canadian and foreign students/residents. To receive student/resident rate, orders must be accompanied by name of affiliated institution, data of term, and the *signature* of program/residency coordinator on institution letterhead. Orders will be billed at individual rate until proof of status is received. Foreign air speed delivery is included in all *Clinics* subscription prices. All prices are subject to change without notice. **POSTMASTER:** Send address changes to *Critical Care Nursing Clinics of North America*, Elsevier Health Sciences Division, Subscription Customer Service, 3251 Riverport Lane, Maryland Heights, MO 63043. **Customer Service: 1-800-654-2452 (US and Canada); 314-447-8871 (outside US and Canada). Fax: 314-447-8029. E-mail: JournalsCustomerService-usa@elsevier.com (for print support) and JournalsOnlineSupport-usa@elsevier.com (for online support).**

Reprints. For copies of 100 or more of articles in this publication, please contact the Commercial Reprints Department, Elsevier Inc., 360 Park Avenue South, New York, New York, 10010-1710; Tel.: (212) 633-3813, Fax: (212) 462-1935, and E-mail: reprints@elsevier.com.

Critical Care Nursing Clinics of North America is covered in *MEDLINE/PubMed (Index Medicus), International Nursing Index, Nursing Citation Index, Cumulative Index to Nursing and Allied Health Literature,* and *RNdex Top 100.*

Printed and bound by CPI Group (UK) Ltd, Croydon, CR0 4YY

Transferred to Digital Print 2012

Contributors

CONSULTING EDITOR

JANET FOSTER, PhD, RN, CNS
Texas Woman's University, College of Nursing, Houston, Texas

GUEST EDITOR

SUSAN MACE WEEKS, DNP, RN, CNS, LMFT, FAAN
Associate Dean, TCU Harris College of Nursing and Health Sciences; Director, TCU
Center for Evidence Based Practice and Research: A Collaborating Center of the
Joanna Briggs Institute, Fort Worth, Texas

AUTHORS

ALICIA C. HAWLEY BARKER, LMSW
Transitional Housing Coordinator, Hope's Door Inc. Domestic Violence Agency, Plano,
Texas

YOLANDA BONE, RN, BSN, CCRN
Adjunct Professor, College of Nursing, Critical Care, South University, Tampa Campus,
Tampa, Florida

DEBORAH BOROWSKE, DNP, MSN, RN, GCNS-BC
Director, Community Health, Geriatrics, Hospice and Home Health, Southwest General
Health Center, Middleburg Heights; Adjunct Faculty, Kent State College of Nursing,
Kent State University, Kent, Ohio

BARBARA CALDWELL, PhD, APN
Professor, Graduate Programs PhD, MSN; Director of Faculty and Scholarly
Development—Acute & Continuum of Care, Graduate Programs; Psychiatric-Mental
Health Nurse Practitioner, Adult Focus MSN Program, School of Nursing, University of
Medicine & Dentistry of New Jersey, Newark, New Jersey

E. RENEE CANTWELL, DNP, RN, CNE
Assistant Professor, New Jersey Center for Evidence Based Practice, University of
Medicine and Dentistry of New Jersey School of Nursing, Newark, New Jersey

REBECCA COFFEY, MSN, CNP
Department of Critical Care Trauma and Burns, Department of Surgery, The Ohio State
University, Columbus, Ohio

CAROLE FARLEY-TOOMBS, RN, MS, CNS, NEA-BC
Director of Clinical Operations for Acute Psychiatric Services, Strong Behavioral Health;
Associate Director of Nursing Practice, Strong Memorial Hospital, University of
Rochester Medical Center, Rochester, New York

VANESSA GENUNG, PhD, RN, PMH-NP-BC, LCSW-ACP, LMFT, LCDC
Wilson School of Nursing, Midwestern State University, Wichita Falls, Texas

DIANE A. HAWLEY, PhD, RN, CCNS, CNE
Associate Professor of Professional Practice, Harris College of Nursing and Health
Sciences, Texas Christian University, Fort Worth, Texas

CHERYL HOLLY, EdD, RN
Associate Professor and Chair, Department of Capacity Building Systems; Director,
New Jersey Center for Evidence Based Practice, University of Medicine and Dentistry of
New Jersey School of Nursing, Newark, New Jersey.

DOLORES M. HUFFMAN, RN, PhD
School of Nursing, Purdue University Calumet, Hammond, Indiana

YURI JADOTTE, MD
Research Associate, New Jersey Center for Evidence Based Practice, University of
Medicine and Dentistry of New Jersey School of Nursing, Newark, New Jersey

SUSAN KAISER, PMHCNS, BC CARN-AP LADC
Associated Clinic of Psychology, Brooklyn Center; Family Life Center, Coon Rapids,
Minnesota

ANNE M. KLEVAY, RN, MSN, PMHCNS-BC
Clinical Nurse Specialist in Psychiatry, Stanford Hospital and Clinics, Stanford,
California

MARY E. LOUGH, RN, PhD, CNS, CCRN, CNRN, CCNS
Critical Care Clinical Nurse Specialist, Stanford Hospital and Clinics, Stanford; Clinical
Professor, Department of Physiological Nursing, School of Nursing, University of
California–San Francisco, San Francisco, California

CLAIRE V. MURPHY, PharmD, BCPS
Department of Pharmacy, The Ohio State University Medical Center; Assistant
Professor, The Ohio State University, Columbus, Ohio

KATHLEEN L. PATUSKY, MA, PhD, RN, CNS
Assistant Professor, Graduate Programs DNP, MSN; Psychiatric-Mental Health Nurse
Practitioner, Adult Focus MSN Program, School of Nursing, University of Medicine &
Dentistry of New Jersey, Newark, New Jersey

LESLIE RITTENMEYER, RN, PsyD, CNE
Professor, School of Nursing, Purdue University Calumet, Hammond, Indiana; Deputy
Director of Evidence Synthesis, Indiana Center for Evidence Based Nursing Practice: A
Collaborating Centre of the Joanna Briggs Institute, Adelaid, Australia

BRUCE RUCK, PharmD, DABAT
Adjunct Faculty, School of Nursing; New Jersey Poison Information and Education
System, New Jersey Medical School, University of Medicine & Dentistry of New Jersey,
Newark, New Jersey

GEORGE BYRON SMITH, DNP, ARNP, GNP-BC
Assistant Professor, College of Nursing, Psychiatric-Mental Health Nursing, South
University, Tampa Campus, Tampa, Florida

DAVID UNKLE, MSN, RN, APN, FCCM
Assistant Professor, Graduate Programs MSN; Assistant Dean for Clinical Affairs &
Coordinator, Acute/Critical Care Nurse Practitioner Program, School of Nursing,
University of Medicine & Dentistry of New Jersey, Newark, New Jersey

Contents

High-dependency environments are complex both from the standpoint of diversity of patient types and the nature of their functioning. Owing to variability in the characteristics of the patient population, the critical care environment presents its own unique set of safety challenges. This article addresses two of those: risk of in-hospital (outside the psychiatric unit) suicide and potential for family or patient aggression. Being attuned not only to the physical status of the patient but also to the emotional/psychological status is paramount in maintaining a safe environment. Staff training and education are paramount in reducing risk.

The treatment of psychiatric issues must be undertaken concurrently with that of acute and critical medical disorders. Too often behavioral symptoms can interfere with patient care. Critical care nurses can provide optimum care only if they are prepared to address psychopathologies that present or emerge from a variety of sources.

The intensive care unit and the inpatient psychiatry unit are different clinical worlds that share patient populations and challenges. In this article, D'Amour's collaborative model is used to analyze interprofessional and interorganizational collaboration between critical care and psychiatry within a single academic medical center.

The overall objective of this meta-aggregate systematic review was to appraise and synthesize the best available evidence on how professional nurses working in hospital environments experience ethical/moral distress. This review considered qualitative research whose participants were professional nurses working in hospital environments and experienced either moral or ethical distress as a result of their patient care responsibilities. Health care institutions need to address concerns related to moral distress by providing structures of support. This support should include education and allow nurses to express ethical concerns and provide nursing care that does not violate their core professional values.

Clients with psychiatric illness are not uncommon to the critical care environment. Often times delirium may be inaccurately attributed to psychosis. Negative perceptions of psychiatric clients may cloud nursing assessment and judgment adversely impacting the outcome for the client. Through education nurses can gain a better understanding of the differences between delirium and psychosis.

Every day, intensive care unit nurses care for critically ill, elderly patients who have not been offered the option of hospice care. With hospice's introduction to the United States in the 1970s, a movement to improve overmedicalization and institutionalization of care for the dying emerged. Despite the steady growth in hospice utilization, many prospective enrollees are not offered the comprehensive comfort care that is a cornerstone of hospice; many are referred late or not at all. Of enrolled patients, more than one third die within 7 days of enrollment.

Substance abuse and dependence require treatment in various acute care settings. Critical care nurses are in a position to assess and initiate knowledge-based best practice strategies for prevention, education, treatment, and rehabilitation referral. This article focuses on increasing the knowledge base of critical care nurses and advanced practice registered nurses and on the neurobiology and current treatments of substances of addiction. Mesolimbic dopamine system (MDS) pathophysiology and neurotransmitter vulnerabilities are identified. The mechanism of action in the MDS for drugs of dependence is explored. Emerging drugs of choice are represented. Evidence-based treatments and levels of care are presented.

Delirium, a common condition seen in hospitalized elderly, can go unrecognized and untreated, contributing to increased morbidity, mortality, length of stay, and cost. Because failure to both recognize and differentiate delirium leaves the patient untreated, there are compelling social, clinical, and financial reasons to improve the identification and prevention of patients with delirium.

The stigma associated with psychiatric and substance abuse disorders is a formidable barrier for persons carrying such a diagnosis or exhibiting symptoms. Nurses' and treatment providers' attitudes can negatively impact the therapeutic process and development of trust necessary for good patient outcomes. Understanding the components of stigma can help nurses to reduce its impact in clinical care settings. Implementing interventions based on the core values of the nurse–patient relationship to enhance understanding, mutual trust, and acceptance of differences can contribute to improved communication and patient assessments in an effort to improve patient outcomes.

THE CLINICS ARE NOW AVAILABLE ONLINE!

Access your subscription at:
www.theclinics.com

Preface

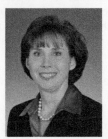

Susan Mace Weeks, DNP, RN, CNS, LMFT
Guest Editor

Sudoku Thinking. Have you ever worked on the solution to a Sudoku puzzle only to find yourself frustrated as you realized the numbers you've entered in one square don't work when combined with the numbers entered in another square? The frustration one experiences when facing a confusing Sudoku puzzle is miniscule when compared with the frustration one experiences when realizing the solution for one aspect of a patient's condition creates a complication for another aspect of a patient's situation. Another type of frustration arises when the desired solution for a particular illness can't be utilized because it is contraindicated by a competing illness. This type of frustration is commonly experienced by critical care nurses caring for patients with mental health and/or addiction issues.

This issue of *Critical Care Nursing Clinics of North America* has been designed to serve as a resource for critical care clinicians facing those frustrations. There are resources for dealing with patients contemplating suicide, addiction issues, delirium syndromes, domestic violence, end-of-life issues, and other combinations of critical care and mental health issues. The overall theme of the issue is the need to understand the interplay of coexisting disease processes and psychosocial complexities. Strategies to improve the care for these patients are presented along with methods to access helpful resources.

The strategies needed to solve a Sudoku puzzle successfully are similar to strategies needed to solve complex, competing patient needs. Those strategies include an awareness of how the solution to one situation will impact a coexisting situation, disciplining oneself to think constantly about the unintended consequences of our treatment plan, identifying and using peers from various disciplines as sounding boards and solution generators, and sharing successful strategies with our professional colleagues. These strategies will increase the likelihood of successfully solving a Sudoku puzzle, but much more importantly, these strategies will increase the likelihood of providing patient-centered, holistic care to the individuals for whom we care.

In closing, I would like to thank many individuals who have assisted me with my role as guest editor of this edition. Dr Jan Foster, consulting editor for *Critical Care Nursing Clinics of North America*, was kind enough to provide me with this opportunity. Katie

Crit Care Nurs Clin N Am 24 (2012) xi–xii
doi:10.1016/j.ccell.2012.01.010
0899-5885/12/$ – see front matter © 2012 Elsevier Inc. All rights reserved.

Hartner, *Clinics* editor, has been an ongoing source of information and guidance throughout the process. The authors who have provided articles for this edition have each been willing to contribute their wisdom, experience, and passion to bring this edition to fruition. I am grateful for the contribution of each individual. My hope is that this edition will improve the care our patients receive as we respond to their unique needs.

Susan Mace Weeks, DNP, RN, CNS, LMFT
TCU Harris College of Nursing and Health Sciences
TCU Center for Evidence Based Practice and Research:
A Collaborating Center of the Joanna Briggs Institute
TCU Box 298620
Fort Worth, TX 76129, USA

E-mail address:
s.weeks@tcu.edu

Effects of Alcohol Use and Abuse on Critically Ill Burn Patients

Rebecca Coffey, MSN, CNP[a],*, Claire V. Murphy, PharmD, BCPS[b,c]

KEYWORDS

- Alcohol abuse • Alcohol withdrawal
- Medication management • Critically ill burn patient

EPIDEMIOLOGY OF BURN INJURY AND ALCOHOL USE

In the United States, approximately 450,000 people are burned every year, with 45,000 injuries severe enough to require hospitalization. The American Burn Association has defined major burns as burns that render the victims critically ill or are associated with inhalational injury and require admission to a specialized burn treatment center or an intensive care unit, with fluid resuscitation an important part of patient care. Major burns account for approximately 12% of all U.S. hospital admissions due to burns.[1] Bard and colleagues[2] stated that alcohol use has been linked to 64% of burn and fire injuries. Furthermore, about 50% of the adult burn patients admitted to U.S. hospitals have either a positive blood or urine alcohol level at the time of burn injury or a history of alcohol abuse, and these rates are anticipated to increase over the next few years.[3,4] In addition to age, increasing burn size, and the existence of inhalation injury, preexisting medical conditions including alcohol abuse increase the mortality associated with burns as well as the length of hospital stay and health care costs.[2–5] The National Burn Repository (NBR) is a voluntary reporting database for burn centers throughout the United States. Thombs and colleagues,[6] using data from 31,338 adult burn patients in the NBR database, found that alcohol abuse was associated with a 1.8-fold higher risk of mortality and increased length of stay among burn survivors. Furthermore, complications after burn surgery increased two- to fivefold from the effects of alcohol on cardiac cells, the immune system, platelet function, splanchnic blood flow, and the pulmonary system.[7] Of note, patients

[a] Department of Critical Care Trauma and Burns, Department of Surgery, The Ohio State University, 410 West 10th Avenue, Columbus, OH 43210, USA
[b] Department of Pharmacy, The Ohio State University Medical Center, 410 West 10th Avenue, Columbus, OH 43210, USA
[c] The Ohio State University, Columbus, OH, USA
* Corresponding author. Division of Critical Care Trauma and Burns, Department of Surgery, The Ohio State University, 410 West 10th Avenue, Columbus, OH 43210.
E-mail address: Rebecca.Coffey@osumc.edu

Crit Care Nurs Clin N Am 24 (2012) 1–7
doi:10.1016/j.ccell.2011.12.001
0899-5885/12/$ – see front matter © 2012 Elsevier Inc. All rights reserved.

who were intoxicated at the time of their burn injury were more likely to have more severe injuries, with larger and deeper burns, and more likely to have inhalation injury.[3(p784)]

DEFINITION OF ALCOHOL USE DISORDERS AND ALCOHOL TOLERANCE

The definition of alcohol use disorders is based on the following diagnostic criteria in the *Diagnostic and Statistical Manual of Mental Health Disorders,* Fourth Edition (DSM-IV)[8]: a maladaptive pattern of alcohol abuse leading to clinically significant impairment or distress, as manifested by one or more of the following, occurring within a 12-month period:

- Recurrent alcohol use resulting in failure to fulfill major role obligations at work, school, or home (eg, repeated absences or poor work performance related to substance use; substance-related absences, suspensions, or expulsions from school; or neglect of children or household)
- Recurrent alcohol use in situations in which it is physically hazardous (eg, driving an automobile or operating a machine)
- Recurrent alcohol-related legal problems (eg, arrests for alcohol-related disorderly conduct)
- Continued alcohol use despite persistent or recurrent social or interpersonal problems caused or exacerbated by the effects of the alcohol (eg, arguments with spouse about consequences of intoxication or physical fights).

The following is the DSM-IV revised[8] definition of alcohol dependence: A maladaptive pattern of alcohol use, leading to clinically significant impairment or distress, as manifested by three or more of the following seven criteria, occurring at any time in the same 12-month period:

1. Tolerance, as defined by either of the following:

   ○ A need for markedly increased amounts of alcohol to achieve intoxication or desired effect
   ○ Markedly diminished effect with continued use of the same amount of alcohol

2. Withdrawal, as defined by either of the following:

   ○ The characteristic withdrawal syndrome for alcohol (refer to DSM-IV for further details)
   ○ Taking alcohol to relieve or avoid withdrawal symptoms

3. Alcohol is often taken in larger amounts or over a longer period than was intended.

4. There is a persistent desire or there are unsuccessful efforts to cut down or control alcohol use.

5. A great deal of time is spent in activities necessary to obtain alcohol, use alcohol, or recover from its effects.

6. Important social, occupational, or recreational activities are given up or reduced because of alcohol use.

7. Alcohol use is continued despite knowledge of having a persistent or recurrent physical or psychological problem that is likely to have been caused or exacerbated by the alcohol (eg, continued drinking despite recognition that an ulcer was made worse by alcohol consumption).

IMPACT OF ALCOHOL ON MULTISYSTEM ORGAN FAILURE

Alcohol intoxication contributes to the potential for multisystem failure in critically ill burn patients. Kavanaugh and colleagues[9] demonstrated that in rats, acute alcohol ingestion before burn injury increased intestinal bacterial translocation and was associated with a loss of both T cells and dendritic cells in the intestine and alterations in intestinal permeability. Alcohol has been shown to have suppressive effects on the immune system and consequently to increase the risk of infection. As major burn patients already experience an overwhelming immune response and a high risk of infection, alcohol dependency can further complicate the intensive care stay, with an increased incidence of sepsis and septic shock.[10]

ALCOHOL AND MAJOR BURN EFFECTS ON ALL BODY SYSTEMS

Al-Sanouri and colleagues described the critical complications of alcohol abuse, listing neurologic, respiratory, gastrointestinal, metabolic, renal, and cardiovascular complications.[11] The neurologic effects of alcohol, including alcohol withdrawal syndrome and hepatic encephalopathy coupled with the fluid shifts from burn shock and possible hypoxia from smoke inhalation or carbon monoxide poisoning, can make it difficult to assess the neurologic status of burn patients. Chronic alcohol abuse has been associated with increased incidence of adult respiratory distress syndrome and more severe multiorgan dysfunction.[12(pS207)] Ventilation and oxygenation in the resuscitation phase present challenges for critical care nurses. Smoke inhalation; exposure to the byproducts of combustion; inhalation of toxic chemicals; and burns of the pulmonary system, neck, and face all contribute to the respiratory complications from burn injury. Furthermore, intubation and mechanical ventilation in burn patients make them more susceptible to pneumonia and increase mortality by 40%.[13] Gastrointestinal (GI) effects of chronic alcohol abuse include gastritis, GI bleeding, and cirrhosis. The burn effects on the GI system include Curling's ulcer, bleeding, and decreased motility of the gut.[11,13] The immune response related to burn injury includes inflammation and the release of prostaglandins and cytokines in the local burn wound. The activation of the hypothalamic–pituitary–adrenal (HPA) axis causes the systemic response of increase oxygen consumption and an increase in the metabolic rate and protein catabolism, causing a decrease in the lean body mass. The preexisting malnutrition associated with alcohol dependency in tandem with the malnutrition and protein catabolism associated with major burn injuries has a significant impact on burn wound healing. The endocrine response includes an increase in catecholamines, cortisol, and glucagon. Metabolic derangements common to patients with alcohol abuse and burn patients include hypokalemia, hypomagnesemia, decreased calcium, decreased phosphorus, hypoglycemia and hyperglycemia, and lactic acidosis.[11,13] Poorly resuscitated or burn patients with resuscitation delays can be susceptible to acute renal failure, and in cases of alcohol abuse nurses must be vigilant in their assessment for renal failure. Retrospective studies of intoxicated burn patients have shown that critically ill burns (those requiring fluid resuscitation or with inhalation injury) are more difficult to resuscitate, with more episodes of hypotension and more operative procedures and hospital-acquired infections.[3] Finally, the effects of alcohol and burn injury on the cardiovascular system include dysrhythmias and tachycardia. Electrolyte imbalances and the hypermetabolic state contribute to the cardiovascular effects.[11,13] In summary, the burn injury and chronic alcohol abuse or alcohol dependency can affect all of the body systems, making the care of these patients challenging for critical care nurses.

Alcohol abuse confounds the recognized standard of care for patients with major burns and full-thickness wounds. Burn care protocols often include early surgical debridement to minimize risk of infection. Burn patients with alcohol withdrawal symptoms may have surgical delays of up to 7 to 10 days, until the withdrawal symptoms abate. These delays significantly increase burn wound complications and the risk for infection and sepsis.[2]

Ingestion of alcohol acutely inhibits the excitatory N-methyl-D-aspartate (NMDA) receptors and activation of inhibitory γ-aminobutyric acid type A (GABA-A) receptors during alcohol ingestion, leading to sedation and anxiolysis. These effects, coupled with burn injury and the inability to protect oneself, result in deeper and larger burns and higher rates of smoke inhalation.[2,14] With chronic alcohol use, the GABA-A receptor function is decreased and the NMDA receptors are up-regulated. When the alcohol is no longer present, the excitatory NMDA function is increased and the inhibition by the GABA-A mechanisms is reduced. This leads to autonomic and neuronal hyperexcitability and the associated clinical manifestations of alcohol withdrawal.[14]

When a burn patient who drinks alcohol is admitted to the critical care unit, alcohol withdrawal syndrome can occur. This constellation of symptoms occurs when a person abruptly stops drinking or diminishes alcohol consumption; it may occur 6 to 24 hours after consumption stops, with symptoms ranging from mild to severe. Critically ill burn patients are placed on narcotic and anxiolytic continuous drips for pain and anxiety control, which may mask the symptoms. The majority of patients who go through alcohol withdrawal syndrome (AWS) experience mild symptoms as a result of autonomic hyperactivity and increased levels of catechloamines.[14] These symptoms can include tremors, nausea, vomiting, anxiety, mild agitation, tachycardia, hypertension, and paroxysmal sweats typically starting within 6 hours of alcohol cessation and peaking within 24 to 48 hours. Severe symptoms can include alcoholic hallucinosis, tonic–clonic seizures, and delirium tremens (DTs).[15] About 30% of patients will experience alcoholic hallucinosis. This syndrome is associated with primarily visual and tactile hallucinations that occur within 8 to 48 hours after alcohol cessation/reduction and last between 1 and 6 days. Tactile hallucinations may include fornication, which can result in excoriation of skin that could be detrimental to wound healing in burn injury. Seizures associated with alcohol withdrawal are usually brief tonic–clonic seizures with onset 12 to 48 hours after the last drink and can occur in up to 10% of patients. Approximately 5% of patients will develop DTs, which are distinguished from alcoholic hallucinosis by the lack of a clear sensorium. DTs occur typically 48 to 72 hours after the last drink, and are associated with delirium, autonomic hyperactivity, and hallucinations.[14] Based on the pathophysiology of DTs, there is also an associated hypermetabolic rate that could potentially have an additive effect with the hypermetabolism associated with burn injury, possibly contributing further to morbidity and mortality. Patients with previous withdrawal are at higher risk for severe symptoms associated with AWS.[2,14]

Management of AWS in critically ill burn patients consists of identification of high-risk patients, prevention, and supportive care. In the critically ill patient with a major burn, alcohol dependency, abuse, or withdrawal may be difficult to assess. These patients may have an unknown history of alcohol use or altered mental status from smoke inhalation, carbon monoxide poisoning, or medications at the time of admission, making it difficult to obtain an accurate history. Because of the difficulties in obtaining a reliable history, studies have focused on alternative objective methods for predicting severity of withdrawal. Studies evaluating the role of admission ethanol levels have shown conflicting results, limiting their predictive value.[14,16,17]

Table 1		
CIWA-Ar Assessment and Treatment		
CIWA-Ar Score	VS and CIWA-AR frequency	Medications (IVP/PO/NG)
Below 8	Every 4 hours × 6	None
8–14	Every 2 hours	Lorazepam 1 mg
15–20	Every 1 hour	Lorazepam 2 mg
21–30	Every 1 hour	Lorazepam 3 mg
31–45	Every 1 hour	Lorazepam 4 mg
For breakthrough	Every 30 minutes	Lorazepam 1–2 mg

Abbreviations: IVP, intravenous push; NG, nasogastric; PO, per os or orally; VS, vital signs.

Assessment of symptoms associated with AWS has similar limitations within the burn-injured population. In addition, the complex physiologic process related to the burn injury and comorbid conditions can further complicate the recognition of alcohol withdrawal. Symptoms of autonomic hyperactivity typically associated with AWS can also be attributed to burn-related pain, hypermetabolism from burn injury, withdrawal from other substances, or sepsis. In addition, intensive care unit (ICU) delirium due to medications, sleep deprivation, and other causes may cloud the diagnosis of AWS. The Clinical Institute Withdrawal Assessment of Alcohol Scale-revised (CIWA-Ar) is the most widely used tool for the assessment of the severity of alcohol withdrawal symptoms (Table 1).[14,18,19] The CIWA-Ar scoring system assesses 10 signs and symptoms of AWS, with a maximum possible score of 67. Although the CIWA-Ar scoring system is validated in detoxification centers and in noncritically ill patients, it has not been validated for use in critically ill burn patients. In addition, the CIWA-Ar scoring system requires a known history of alcohol use and the ability to communicate with the patient, which limits the applicability of this assessment strategy in this population.

Benzodiazepines are the gold standard for treatment of AWS and work as GABA receptor agonists like alcohol.[14] Although there are no clear data supporting one benzodiazepine over another, the method of administration has been shown to impact outcomes. The two primary options for administration of benzodiazepines for AWS include scheduled dosing and symptom triggered dosing. In symptom-triggered therapy, the CIWA-Ar scale is paired with a sliding scale benzodiazepine regimen with administration of higher doses of benzodiazepines with increasing severity of withdrawal. The goal of treatment is light sedation, and the emphasis is on accurate assessment of patients' withdrawal symptoms and then adequate dosing with benzodiazepines based on the assessment of severity of the AWS.[20] Despite the favorable outcomes with this approach, this method relies on the CIWA-AR scoring system, which has limited validity in critically ill burn patients.[2,14,18,21,22]

CONCLUSIONS

Burn patients with alcohol abuse or dependency typically have larger burns, a higher risk of inhalation injury, a larger number of complications, a 1.8-fold higher risk of mortality, and increased length of stay among burn survivors.[6] Abuse in critically ill burn patients may be insidious and it is therefore paramount that a careful history and physical be performed on initial examination, including measurement of blood or urine alcohol levels. Obtaining a detailed history of alcohol abuse for critically ill burn patients, the inclusion of alcohol withdrawal assessment with all patients who are at risk, and the use of measurements of blood or urine alcohol levels on admission are important in determination of risk and early recognition of alcohol withdrawal. The ever vigilant critical care nurse can recognize the effects of alcohol withdrawal early, and coupled with a physical examination and history, can tailor the treatment for the best outcomes. It is important to involve the social worker and psychologist early so that appropriate referrals can be made. The nurse practitioner, bedside nurse, and pharmacist are critical members of the multidisciplinary team and can make essential contributions to the development, monitoring, implementation, and evaluation of the treatment of alcohol withdrawal in patients with major burns.

REFERENCES

1. American Burn Association. Burn incidences and treatment in the United States: 2011 fact sheet. Available at: http://www.ameribur.org/resources_factsheet.php. Accessed October 8, 2011.
2. Bard MR, Goettler CE, Toschlog EA, et al. Alcohol withdrawal syndrome: turning minor injuries into a major problem. J Trauma Inj Infect Crit Care 2006;61:1441–6.
3. Silver GM, Albright JM, Schermer CR, et al. Adverse clinical outcomes associated with elevated blood alcohol levels at the time of burn injury. J Burn Care Res 2008;29: 784–9.
4. Holmes WJ, Hold P, James MI. The increasing trend in alcohol-related burns: its impact on a tertiary burn centre. Burns 2009;36:938–43.
5. Coffey R, Kulisek J, Tanda R, et al. Impact of the implementation of an alcohol withdrawal guideline on patients with burn injuries. Clin Nurse Spec 2011;25(6): 286–93.
6. Thombs BD, Singh VA, Halonen J, et al. The effects of preexisting medical comorbidities on mortality and length of hospital stay in acute burn injury. Evidence from a national sample of 31,338 adult burn patients. Ann Surg 2007;245:629–34.
7. Choudhry MA, Ba ZF, Rana SN, et al. Alcohol ingestion before burn injury decreases splanchnic blood flow and oxygen delivery. Am J Physiol Heart Circ Physiol 2005;288: 716–21.
8. American Psychiatric Association. Diagnostic and statistical manual of mental disorders. 4th revised edition. Washington, DC: American Psychiatric Association; 2000.
9. Kavanaugh MK, Clark C, Goto M. Effect of acute alcohol ingestion prior to burn injury on intestinal bacterial growth and barrier function. Burns 2005;31:290–6.
10. O'Brien JM Jr, Lu B, Ali NA, et al. Alcohol dependence is independently associated with sepsis, septic shock, and hospital mortality among adult intensive care unit patients. Crit Care Med 2007;35:345–50.
11. Al-Sanouri I, Dikin M, Soubani AO. Critical care aspects of alcohol abuse. South Med J 2005;98:374–81.
12. Moss M, Burnham EL. Chronic alcohol abuse, acute respiratory distress syndrome and multiple organ dysfunction. Crit Care Med 2003;31(Suppl):S207–12.
13. Herndon DN. Total Burn Care. 3rd edition. Philadelphia: Elsevier Health Sciences; 2007.
14. Sarff M, Gold JA. Alcohol withdrawal syndromes in the intensive care unit. Crit Care Med 2010;38(Suppl 9):S494–501.
15. Bayard M, McIntyre J, Hill KR, et al. Alcohol withdrawal syndrome. Am Fam Physician 2004;69:1443–50.
16. Rathlev NK, Ulrich AS, Fish SS, et al. Clinical characteristics as predictors of recurrent alcohol-related seizures. Acad Emerg Med 2006;7:886–91.
17. Vinson DC, Menezes M. Admission alcohol level: a predictor of the course of alcohol withdrawal. J Fam Pract 1991;33:161–7.

18. Weinberg JA, Magnotti LJ, Fischer PE, et al. Comparison of intravenous ethanol versus diazepam for alcohol withdrawal prophylaxis in the trauma ICU: results of a randomized trial. J Trauma 2008;64:99–104.
19. Keys VA. Alcohol withdrawal during hospitalization. Am J Nurs 2011;111:40–4 [quiz: 45–6].
20. Jaeger TM, Lohr RH, Pankratz VS. Symptom-triggered therapy for alcohol withdrawal syndrome in medical inpatients. Mayo Clin Proc 2001;76:695–701.
21. Daeppenn JB, Burnand B, Schnyder C, et al. Validation of the addiction severity index in French speaking alcoholic patients. J Stud Alcohol 1996;57:585–90.
22. Saitz R, Palfai TP, Cheng DM, et al. Brief intervention for medical inpatients with unhealthy alcohol use: a randomized controlled trial. Ann Intern Med 2007;146:167–76.

Psychiatric and Addiction Consultation for Patients in Critical Care

Susan Kaiser, PMHCNS, BC CARN-AP LADC[a,b,*]

KEYWORDS

- Critical care • Addiction • Chemical dependency
- Comorbidity • Dual diagnosis • Consultation
- Collaboration

Chemical dependency, otherwise termed addiction, is a complex medical, psychological, and spiritual illness.[1] The ubiquitous presence of chemical dependency/addiction's impacts other disorders and must be considered in the initial intervention and treatment planning. Recent scientific research has determined conclusively that addiction is also a chronic physical disease that damages key parts of the brain: cerebral cortex and limbic system.[2] The progressive effects of addiction include structural and physiologic changes to the brain.[2,3]

A key symptom coinciding with the progression of the addiction disease process is tolerance. Tolerance is the capacity to endure a large amount of substance without adverse effect, showing a decreased sensitivity to subsequent increasing doses of the same substance.[4] Tolerance is listed as a diagnostic criteria of chemical dependency by the *Diagnostic and Statistical Manual of Mental Disorders, Fourth Edition* (DSM-IV).[4] Research on tolerance has occupied a central point in the literature[5–7] since the beginning of study on addiction. The development of tolerance is linked to organic complications,[8] and in recent years research has linked tolerance specifically to features of learning and memory.[5,7]

Kaiser serves as member of panel for the American Nursing Credentialing Center study October 2008 to set the passing score for the ANCC Adult Psychiatric Advanced Nursing Exam for 2009–2010.

The author has nothing to disclose.

[a] 6200 Shingle Creek Parkway, Suite 350, Brooklyn Center, MN 55430, USA

[b] Family Life Center, 1930 Coon Rapids Boulevard, Coon Rapids, MN 55433, USA

* Corresponding author. Family Life Center, 1930 Coon Rapids Boulevard, Coon Rapids, MN 55433.

E-mail address: skkaiser@msn.com

LITERATURE REVIEW
Chemical Dependency

It is estimated that 30% to 50% of all patients admitted to a hospital have alcohol misuse related factors[9] and 18% to 20% of patients seen in ambulatory settings have alcohol abuse/dependency problems.[10] The Department of Health and Human Services states that nearly 17 million Americans meet the diagnostic criteria for alcoholism, and 2 million Americans suffer from alcohol-related liver disease, including alcoholic hepatitis and cirrhosis.[11] The long-term effects of alcohol dependency on the brain have been most studied. Organic consequences of alcoholism are many, and may include alcoholic dementia, among other cognitive deficits.[12]

The 2010 Drug Abuse Warning Network (DAWN) reported that the total number of drug-related emergency department (ED) visits between 2004 and 2009 increased 81%.[13] In the same period, the total number of ED visits involving nonmedical use of pharmaceuticals increased 98.4% (from 627,291 to 1.244,679 visits). The largest increase in use of pharmaceuticals associated with ED visits included oxycodone (242.2% increase), alprazolam (148.3% increase), and hydrocodone products (124.5% increase). Between 2005 and 2009, ED visits involving adverse reactions to pharmaceuticals increased 82.9%, from 1,250,337 to 2,287,273.

It is also stated in the current literature that the diagnosis of addiction is not age specific[14] and occurs in a very wide age range. According to the 2005 Substance Abuse and Mental Health Services Administration (SAMHSA) report to Congress, entitled *National Survey on Drug Abuse and Health*, in 2004, 23 million Americans aged 12 years and older needed specialty treatment for alcohol or illicit drug problems.[15] The DAWN report stated that between 2004 and 2009 patients aged 20 years or younger requesting ED treatment resulting from nonmedical use of pharmaceuticals increased 45.4% (116,644 to169,589 visits respectively).[13] In 2009, 16 million patients aged 12 years and older had taken prescriptive medication for nonmedical purposes at least once in the year before being surveyed.[16] The DAWN report also stated that between 2005 and 2009 ED visits involving adverse reactions to pharmaceuticals were made by patients aged 65 years and older, an increase in this population of 82.9% (1, 250,377 to 2,287,273 visits).[13]

Cychosz asserts that new research data are necessary to evaluate the strong association between drug use and crime. Approximately one-half of interpersonal violence incidences are alcohol related.[17] Understanding the costs to society of criminal behavior helps to establish policies and evaluate drug abuse services.[18] According to this research, the new estimates of crime costs associated with addiction include a total of 13 offenses. One example of these offenses is murder, the most costly crime, with an estimated cost of $8.9 million for 2010. The White House Office on National Drug Control Policy stated that during 1988 to 1995 Americans spent $57.3 billion on illicit drugs.[19] The 2001 Policy report, entitled *The Nation's Number One Problem*, stated that untreated addiction costs America $400 billion a year.[20]

Substance misuse has predictable disease and medical consequences demanding treatment.[21] Inadequate treatment increases the risk for human immunodeficiency virus (HIV), hepatitis B and C, cardiac and pulmonary diseases, suicide, criminalization, unemployment, homelessness, separation from families and communities, malnutrition, compromised immune system, cardiomyopathy, ulcers and esophagitis, altered gonadal function, liver cirrhosis, and cancer.[22,23] These predictable medical and social conditions, associated with chemical dependency/addiction, are often unrecognized and overlooked. Lack of referral and assistance for these medical complications results in serious treatment gaps, which sabotages the patient's efforts to comply, as well as recovery prognosis.[21,24]

Collateral consequences of substance misuse, often not identified, can include relational conflicts, childcare needs, difficulty attending treatment due to childcare needs, and involvement of child protection services.[24]

Psychiatric Disorders

Seven to ten million individuals in the United States have at least one psychiatric disorder as well as an alcohol or drug disorder.[23] Forty-three percent of youth receiving mental health services in the United States have been diagnosed with a co-occurring disorder. Dual diagnosis and co-occurring disorder are terms meaning the occurrence of two disorders at the same time.[25] According to the 1999 report from the Department of Health and Human Services, individuals experiencing psychiatric disorders and substance abuse disorder simultaneously have greater difficulty seeking and receiving diagnostic and treatment services.[26] The 2002 SAMHSA report concluded that if one of the co-occurring disorders goes untreated, both usually get worse and develop complications.[27]

An individual with a mental health disorder is at increased risk for developing a substance abuse disorder, and conversely, an individual with a substance abuse disorder is at increased risk for developing a mental disorder.[28] Consequently, co-occurring disorders often require high-cost ED care and inpatient treatment. The SAMHSA 2002 report observes that the individuals with co-occurring disorders have lives that have been disrupted by these disorders; enduring lost families and sometimes lost lives.[23]

Alcoholism is now the third leading cause of death in the United States following heart disease and cancer. Although exact statistics for deaths caused by alcohol and drug abuse are not definitive, the number is surely in the tens of thousands per year.[2] These staggering facts/costs are reason to urgently reevaluate current perspectives of chemical dependency, educational requirements for chemical dependency treatment providers, and current treatment methods.

According to the RAND study, every dollar spent on treatment leads to a $7.46 reduction in crime-related spending and lost productivity.[29] In the 2005 Report to Congress on Addictions Treatment Workforce Development, the then Assistant Surgeon General, Eric Broderick, DDS, MPH, stated, "the human, social and economic costs of not treating substance use disorders is indisputable."[30(p2)]

TREATMENT BARRIERS FOR CO-OCCURRING DISORDERS

The 2005 National Survey on Drug Use and Health stated, "substance use treatment centers have inadequate infrastructure to support current and future demands for treatment."[15(p412-6)] The report further noted this inadequacy in existing infrastructure because of the following citations:

1. There exists significant social stigma attached to the diagnosis of chemical dependency, to those treated for this disease, and to those treating the co-occurring disorders.[24,31]
2. There exists a lack of a common standard for educational preparation for those providing the treatment (nursing and medical).[24] These various levels of educational preparation create treatment gaps and lack of consensus about treatment. with minimal consensus about: "priority of diagnosis in treatment, treatment priorities, which results in inconsistent treatment practice patterns."[12]

3. Varying licensure and staffing requirements results in inconsistent treatment practices and treatment models.[23] In addition to varying credentials and treatment philosophies, salaries also vary, affecting recruitment and retention.[23] Thus, individuals with co-occurring mental health and substance abuse disorders must negotiate treatment without treatment system common standards for care.
4. The lack of provision of integrated treatment ranges across a continuum from excellent/holistic to minimal/incompetent.[15]

Historically, the clinical setting also evidences adversity to addressing the chemical dependency diagnosis.[32] There exists an adversity by clinical providers to address the addiction diagnosis with patients. According to a landmark national study about the treatment of alcoholism, 82% of doctors admitted avoiding addressing the clinical evidence of alcoholism with their patients.[33] This would imply a gross pattern of ignoring treatment needs of patients as the tolerance level to substances actively progress. It is a common occurrence that the chemical dependency diagnosis is not found on diagnostic Axis I, regardless of significant historical evidence of previous chemical dependency symptoms/diagnosis/treatment. It is not uncommon, in the practice setting, to find patient's being treated for dual diagnosis[25] also provided tolerance-developing medication, which is contraindicated in the treatment of chemical dependency. These same patients may also experience easy access to tolerance-developing prescriptive medication for complaints of pain and anxiety. This occurs without prescriptive medication trials using nontolerance developing medication options.[12] These same patients presenting prescription-induced opioid withdrawal symptoms usually cannot be convinced they have developed tolerance with heightened sensitivity to pain.[2] Often these patients perceive efforts to interrupt the prescription-induced tolerance as destructive.[2] There are circumstances when use of opioids is indicated. However, the decision to do so should be with consideration of the chemical dependency diagnosis and include a plan for long-term pain management using nontolerance inducing medication options, whenever possible.[12,31] Also, there is reason for concern that prescriptive-seeking behaviors are for diversion of the medications.

According to Nora Volkow, MD, Director of the National Institute of Drug Abuse (NIDA), despite recent scientific advances explaining that addiction is a disease that affects both brain and behavior; many people today do not understand why individuals become addicted to drugs or how drugs change the brain to foster compulsive behavior.[34]

EDUCATIONAL DEFICIT

Although the diagnosis of chemical dependency is a significant component of so many ED treatment requests and other forms of urgent medical care needs, a national survey of 335 nursing schools found that 72% devoted less then 5 hours of total curriculum to the disease of chemical dependency.[35] The physiology of addiction, and treatment principles, are not a required competency in the educational preparation for nurses.[36] Chemical dependency is often missing from curriculum requirements for high-level practitioners, or may be relegated to notable mention in the overall curriculum.[37,38]

The SAMHSA 2002 report recommends:

1. Improved screening and assessment to identify individuals with co-occurring substance abuse disorders and mental disorders. This recommendation includes understanding that persons with dual diagnosis often use denial and do not enter the system to request help easily. When aid is requested, the mental health

disorder may be masked by substance abuse, complicating assessment and diagnosis. Such a challenging presentation requires specialized assessment and treatment planning.

2. Integrated treatment programs are recommended, requiring interaction between mental health and substance abuse clinicians in the form of consultation and collaboration. The evidence base is growing about the effectiveness of interventions, which include individual treatment plans based on the individual's stage of recovery; therapeutic relationship; medication management; and referrals for other basic needs, such as housing and employment, to facilitate treatment.

3. Integrated organizational structure to ensure adequate treatment and easy access for other services to meet all the patient's basic needs.

4. Integrated system providing an organizational structure support for treatment of co-occurring substance abuse disorders. The system is responsible for: appropriate funding necessary to support the continuum of services indicated, credentialing and licensing standards, needs assessment, planning, and other related functions.[23]

TREATMENT REQUIREMENT

Establishment of treatment protocol and practice collaboration between treatment specialties is necessary to remedy these treatment gaps and improve treatment outcomes. Adoption of best practice standards would require a stable infrastructure, organizational commitment, and staff development.[30]

EVIDENCE-BASED RECOMMENDATIONS

According to Harkness and Bower, the presence of mental health workers on-site in primary care resulted in significant reduction of primary care providers' need for consultation, rates of psychotropic prescribing, prescribing costs, and rates of mental health referrals.[32] This evidence supports the assertion that request by critical care specialists for consultation with chemical dependency and mental health nursing specialists would result in improved response to treatment, greater survival rates, and reduced social costs:

1. Integration of specialty skills and referral/consultation between specialties results in more holistic care.[39]

2. Nursing practice is oriented toward holistic treatment, and nursing specialists in addiction/mental health would practice holistically, recognizing and providing for the full scope of patient needs.[40]

3. In the practice of recognizing and affirming social, emotional, and spiritual needs at all levels of patient care, medical status is positively impacted.[37]

4. Human needs are not isolated and compartmentalized, but rather integrated and interdependent. No single treatment is appropriate for all persons.[2,41,42]

CONTRIBUTION OF CREDENTIALED TREATMENT PROVIDERS FOR CONSULTATION IN CRITICAL CARE

There are various levels of credentialed medical/psychiatric, chemical dependency specialists appropriate for critical care of psychiatric and addicted patients.

1. Addictionologists and psychiatrists are board certified medical doctors specializing in addiction or psychiatric treatment. The scope of practice of the medical doctor with board certification includes specialties if addiction or psychiatry is diagnostic, critical care, and treatment director. The medical specialist is the

treatment team leader. A board-certified addictionolgist or psychiatrist can be located through the state board of medical practitioners or via referral.

2. A certified addiction/psychiatric registered nurse–advanced practice (CARN–AP) (PMHCNS–BC) is a registered nurse who has obtained a master's degree in nursing science with specialized/credentialed scope of practice in addiction. The advanced practice nurse would also have a specialty in another area of treatment such as psychiatry. The scope of practice of the master's prepared nurse/ CARN–AP or PMHCNS–BC includes diagnostic, triage, critical and ongoing care, family interventions, and treatment planning and can also serve as treatment team leader.[41]

3. A registered nurse certified in addiction treatment (CARN) has a 2-year college nursing degree (AD) or 4-year college nursing degree (BSN). The specialist nurse, generalist level, has board-certified expertise in addiction and as a registered nurse can identify level of risk and contribute to prevention and intervention for patients and their families.[41] The generalist level psychiatric nurse has similar skills in psychiatry or another specialty such as medical/surgical.

Nursing addiction certification is obtained through International Nursing Society on Addiction (IntNSA) located at www.IntNSA.org.

4. In addition, those trained as drug and alcohol counselors are licensed by individual State Board of Behavioral Health, and can be located via chemical dependency departments and treatment centers for alcohol and drug treatment services, or through State Board of Behavioral Health.

There are various official websites for locating addiction treatment centers and obtaining research information. SAMHSA (www.samhsa.gov) publishes a free chemical dependency treatment locator for centers of government-recognized treatment. SAMHSA can be contacted by calling 800-729-668.

ADVANCED NURSING PRACTICE/PSYCHIATRIC DISORDERS/ADDICTION
Critical Care Patient Services

1. Nursing practice is uniquely conformed to the principles of collaborative practice.[12] Nursing practice is differentiated from medicine by designating equal priority to disease prevention and wellness of the whole person. This approach is termed holistic treatment.[43] As cited earlier, according to R. E. Drake, if one of the co-occurring disorders goes untreated, both usually get worse and develop complications.[28] The chemical dependency diagnosis implies need for holistic care because of the extreme effect substance misuse has on psychosocial and general health status. The advanced practice nurse with addiction certification and psychiatric certification is capable of identifying the condition of dual diagnosis and understanding the overlapping symptoms of drug addiction and mental illness. Accurate assessment and comprehensive treatment (planning) is crucial to ensure best and most cost effective outcome. Surveys show a high rate of comorbidity between drug addiction and other mental illnesses.[25]

The scope of practice for master's prepared nurse with psychiatric and addiction certification includes[41]:

- Initiation of the therapeutic relationship.
- Providing addiction screening, psychiatric *and* chemical dependency diagnosis for the identified patient. These diagnoses should immediately be incorporated, and prioritized, on diagnostic Axis I.

- Family assessment for identifying the structural aspects of the family communication patterns as they relate to the identified patient's diagnosis.[24]
- Appropriate psychiatric intervention.
- Patient/family education and referrals for treatment and referral to a support group.[44]
- Treatment plan including laboratory tests and medication intervention.
- Treatment team leadership establishing treatment method and priorities. Some of these skills are within the scope of practice for the CARN (Certified Addiction Registered Nurse), including therapeutic relationship, addiction diagnosis, education, and referrals.[44]

2. Collaboration requires time, preparation and supportive structures built on preexisting clinical relationships."[45] System changes must be made at the top of the system, using system education to implement changes. Collaboration between medical/psychiatric and addiction specialists, at all levels, provides comprehensive (holistic) health care services.
3. Communication with the social support system for the critical care patient should also be a part of the mechanism used by the treatment team for treatment planning.[46] The therapeutic purposes of such a meeting would be to gain information essential in treatment planning and to strengthen the patient's social support system. Improving the support level for the patient improves prognosis and treatment outcomes.[47] Information about the identified patient's social and treatment history is useful for:

- Confirming the patient's report
- Assessment of the needs of the patient's support system with appropriate referrals
- Gaining collaborative information about the patient's patterns of use
- Development of a crisis plan
- Development of relapse prevention planning.

4. Contacting 12-step program offices, when appropriate, to ask for a member visit to the hospitalized patient is also appropriate. Monitoring and directing peer level interventions for correlation with treatment goals requires advanced skill. This practice could encourage 12-step referral posthospitalization. Members of 12-step groups can contribute powerful peer-level patient support. A recent study determined that this level of support is very important in influencing entry and retention into alcohol/drug-addiction treatment as well as prognosis.[47]

Psychiatric and chemical dependency intervention in critical care should provide a diagnosis and assessment of the patient's readiness for change with treatment plan oriented toward the individual patient and the patient's support system. Every effort should be extended to establish the critical care patient's commitment to treatment.

CLINICAL EXAMPLE OF CHEMICAL DEPENDENCY TREATMENT BARRIERS

Patient B is age 18, Caucasian, height 6'1', weight 170 lb, body mass index (BMI) 22.4. He has requested evaluation in outpatient psychiatric clinic. Patient B presented with psychiatric symptoms of acute anxiety with evidence of perceptual disturbances. He reported that this anxiety had not responded to the previous medication treatment efforts. He was not taking medications at the time of this appointment. He was vague about treatment history. He came to the appointment with his mother, who also provided transportation. She accompanied him into the evaluation office, was vigilant

Table 1
Adult patient placement criteria for the treatment of psychoactive substance use disorders

Levels of Care Criteria Dimensions	Level I Outpatient Treatment	Level II Intensive Outpatient Treatment	Level III Medically Monitored Intensive Inpatient Treatment	Level IV Medically Managed Intensive Inpatient Treatment
1 Acute intoxication and/or withdrawal potential	No withdrawal risk	Minimal withdrawal risk	Severe withdrawal risk but manageable in Level III	Severe withdrawal risk
2 Biomedical conditions and complications	None or very stable	None or distracting from addiction treatment and manageable in Level II	Requires medical monitoring but not intensive treatment	Requires 24-hour medical, nursing care
3 Emotional/behavioral conditions and complications	None or very stable	Mild severity with potential to distract from recovery	Moderate severity needing a 24-hour structured setting	Severe problems requiring 24-hour psychiatric care with concomitant addiction treatment
4 Treatment acceptance/ resistance	Willing to cooperate but needs motivating and monitoring strategies	Resistance high enough to require structured program, but not so high as to render outpatient treatment ineffective	Resistance high enough despite negative consequences and needs intensive motivating strategies in 24-hour structure	Problems in this dimension do not qualify patient for Level IV treatment

5 Relapse potential	Able to maintain abstinence and recovery goals with minimal support	Intensification of addiction symptoms and high likelihood of relapse without close monitoring and support	Unable to control us despite active participation in less intensive care and needs 24-hour structure	Problems in this dimension do not qualify patient for Level IV treatment
6 Recovery environment	Supportive recovery environment and/ or patient has skills to cope	Environment supportive but with structure and support, the patient can cope	Environment dangerous for recovery necessitating removal from the environment; logistical impediments to outpatient treatment	Problems in this dimension do not qualify patient for Level IV treatment

NOTE: This overview of the Adult Admission Criteria is an approximate summary to illustrate the principal concepts and structure of the criteria.
Source: Hoffman N, Halikas J, Mee-Lee D, et al. Patient placement criteria for the treatment of psychoactive substance use disorders. Washington, DC: American Society of Addiction Medicine.

Patient:_____ Date: _____ Time: _____ (24 hour clock, midnight = 00:00)

Pulse or heart rate, taken for one minute:_____ Blood pressure:_____

NAUSEA AND VOMITING -- Ask "Do you feel sick to your stomach? Have you vomited?" Observation.
 no nausea and no vomiting
 mild nausea with no vomiting

 intermittent nausea with dry heaves

 constant nausea, frequent dry heaves and vomiting

TACTILE DISTURBANCES -- Ask "Have you any itching, pins an needles sensations, any burning, any numbness, or do you feel bugs crawling on or under your skin?" Observation.
0 none
1 very mild itching, pins and needles, burning or numbness
2 mild itching, pins and needles, burning or numbness
3 moderate itching, pins and needles, burning or numbness
4 moderately severe hallucinations
5 severe hallucinations
6 extremely severe hallucinations
7 continuous hallucinations

TREMOR -- Arms extended and fingers spread apart. observation.
 no tremor
 not visible, but can be felt fingertip to fingertip

 moderate, with patient's arms extended

 severe, even with arms not extended

AUDITORY DISTURBANCES -- Ask "Are you more aware of sounds around you? Are they harsh? Do they frighten you? Are you hearing anything that is disturbing to you? Are you hearing things you know are not there?" Observation.
0 not present
1 very mild harshness or ability to frighten
2 mild harshness or ability to frighten
3 moderate harshness or ability to frighten
4 moderately severe hallucinations
5 severe hallucinations
6 extremely severe hallucinations
7 continuous hallucinations

PAROXYSMAL SWEATS -- Observation.
 no sweat visible
 barely perceptible sweating, palms moist

 beads of sweat obvious on forehead

 drenching sweats

VISUAL DISTURBANCES -- Ask "Does the light appear to be too bright? Is its color different? Does it hurt your eyes? Are you seeing anything that is disturbing to you? Are you seeing things you know are not there?" Observation.
0 not present
1 very mild sensitivity
2 mild sensitivity
3 moderate sensitivity
4 moderately severe hallucinations
5 severe hallucinations
6 extremely severe hallucinations
7 continuous hallucinations

ANXIETY -- Ask "Do you feel nervous?" Observation.
 no anxiety, at ease
 mild anxious

 moderately anxious, or guarded, so anxiety is inferred

 equivalent to acute panic states as seen in severe delirium or ute schizophrenic reactions

HEADACHE, FULLNESS IN HEAD -- Ask "Does your head feel different? Does it feel like there is a band around your head?" Do not rate for dizziness or lightheadedness. Otherwise, rate severity.
0 not present
1 very mild
2 mild
3 moderate
4 moderately severe
5 severe
6 very severe
7 extremely severe

Fig. 1. Clinical Institute Withdrawal Assessment of Alcohol Scale, Revised (CIWA-Ar).

about his condition, and voiced concern about her ability to manage him alone during the day while his father was at work. She reported that she had taken a leave of absence form work to provide supervision for her son; otherwise he would be alone at home with potential for harmful outcome in his present psychiatric status.

Patient B sat down in an office chair, next to his mother, but was incapable of answering questions. His eye contact was minimal. He was very restless, and argued with his mother about her response to questions posed. He also was very paranoid, asserting misinterpretation of questions asked. He insisted on focusing on details of social threats experienced in present living circumstances. He demonstrated further agitation in response to his mother's statements, resulting in increased (precombative) agitated status.

His mother further expressed dismay at the fact that when they travel "up north" to their summer cabin, her son would "always be calm." She worried about "having to quit work altogether in order to take him "up north" to live.

Date: _____   Clinic ID# _____   T _____ P _____ R _____ B/P _____

From the time of your previous dose of methadone, please indicate if you are having any of the following withdrawal symptoms by **rating its severity.**						How long **AFTER** your last dose did you begin to feel this symptom?			
								Onset (hrs)	
1	Anxious/Nervous	0	1	2	3	4	3-4 ☐	8 ☐	16 ☐	24 ☐
2	Body Aches & Pains	0	1	2	3	4	3-4 ☐	8 ☐	16 ☐	24 ☐
3	Constipation	0	1	2	3	4	3-4 ☐	8 ☐	16 ☐	24 ☐
4	Diarrhea	0	1	2	3	4	3-4 ☐	8 ☐	16 ☐	24 ☐
5	Drug Hunger/Craving	0	1	2	3	4	3-4 ☐	8 ☐	16 ☐	24 ☐
6	Goosebumps	0	1	2	3	4	3-4 ☐	8 ☐	16 ☐	24 ☐
7	Hot/Cold Flashes	0	1	2	3	4	3-4 ☐	8 ☐	16 ☐	24 ☐
8	Muscle Twitching	0	1	2	3	4	3-4 ☐	8 ☐	16 ☐	24 ☐
9	Nausea	0	1	2	3	4	3-4 ☐	8 ☐	16 ☐	24 ☐
10	Restlessness	0	1	2	3	4	3-4 ☐	8 ☐	16 ☐	24 ☐
11	Runny Nose	0	1	2	3	4	3-4 ☐	8 ☐	16 ☐	24 ☐
12	Sedation/Sleepiness	0	1	2	3	4	3-4 ☐	8 ☐	16 ☐	24 ☐
13	Shaking	0	1	2	3	4	3-4 ☐	8 ☐	16 ☐	24 ☐
14	Stomach Cramps	0	1	2	3	4	3-4 ☐	8 ☐	16 ☐	24 ☐
15	Sweating	0	1	2	3	4	3-4 ☐	8 ☐	16 ☐	24 ☐
16	Teary Eyes	0	1	2	3	4	3-4 ☐	8 ☐	16 ☐	24 ☐
17	Vomiting	0	1	2	3	4	3-4 ☐	8 ☐	16 ☐	24 ☐
18	Yawning	0	1	2	3	4	3-4 ☐	8 ☐	16 ☐	24 ☐

Patient Name (Print) _____ Signature _____ Date: _____
Patient's Current Dose _____mg Dose Adjustment Made _____ New Dose _____mg Effective Date _____
Nurse Signature _____ Date: _____

Fig. 2. Subjective Opiate Withdrawal Scale (SOWS). (*Adapted from* Handelsman L, Cochrane KJ, Aronson MJ, et al. Two new rating scales for opiate withdrawal. Am J Alcohol Abuse 1987;13:293–308.)

It was assessed that an outpatient psychiatric evaluation would be impossible because of the following presenting factors:

- The patent's **unpredictability** and paranoia combined with a high level of agitation and potential for aggression
- Patient B's **inability to interpret the communication accurately,** resulting in increased paranoia and agitation
- **Etiology** of anxiety and paranoia as well as atypical or inverse response to previous medication trials.

A transport hold was completed and the patient was sent to a local ED for further evaluation. In short order, the attending physician requested the ED representative call the referring clinician for additional information. The assessment and symptom presentation was repeated to the hospital representative. The hospital ED caller informed, with opposition, that patient B was quiet and resting at the time with no evidence of these symptoms, although his toxicology had been positive for marijuana. Ultimately, it was learned that patient B was not admitted and no follow-up information was provided.

This scenario is not uncommon. One of the few comprehensible statements this patient made, as he was being loaded onto the ambulance, was that he would not ever come back to the clinic sending him to the hospital ED. This response also is not uncommon. This example evidences diagnostic/practice confusion, lack of effective collaboration with lack of cooperation in the prioritizing needs of the patient and immediate family, and multiple other treatment barriers. The primary differences and disagreement in assessment between clinic provider and hospital ED will most certainly result in:

1. Patient B and his family being less willing to seek help in the future
2. Patient B and his family being less confident in the assessment and treatment process

Date .... Time ....

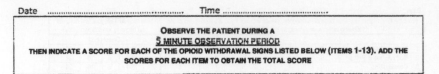

	SIGN	MEASURES		SCORE
1	Yawning	0 = no yawns	1 = ≥ 1 yawn	
2	Rhinorrhoea	0 = < 3 sniffs	1 = ≥ 3 sniffs	
3	Piloerection (observe arm)	0 = absent	1 = present	
4	Perspiration	0 = absent	1 = present	
5	Lacrimation	0 = absent	1 = present	
6	Tremor (hands)	0 = absent	1 = present	
7	Mydriasis	0 = absent	1 = > 3 mm	
8	Hot and Cold flushes	0 = absent	1 = shivering / huddling for warmth	
9	Restlessness	0 = absent	1 = frequent shifts of position	
10	Vomiting	0 = absent	1 = present	
11	Muscle twitches	0 = absent	1 = present	
12	Abdominal cramps	0 = absent	1 = Holding stomach	
13	Anxiety	0 = absent	1 = mild - severe	
	TOTAL SCORE			

Fig. 3. Objective Opioid Withdrawal Scale (OOWS). (*Adapted from* Handelsman L, Cochrane KJ, Aronson MJ, et al. Two new rating scales for opiate withdrawal. Am J Alcohol Abuse 1987;13:293–308.)

3. Patient B and his family being confused about the dynamics of the assessing process, necessitating spending the day in the ED and leading to frustration about the outcome.

In addition, the author submits that the possible reason for difference in mental status in patient B at home and "up north" is the availability of marijuana (and possibly other contraband) supply at home base. Marijuana (tetrahydrocannabinol [THC])[4] withdrawal can most certainly create such psychiatric status of paranoia, agitation, and hallucination, as evidenced in this example. This is especially so in combination with preexisting psychiatric diagnosis (comorbidity) or substance-induced psychotic condition. How could this petite mother, alone, be able to safely manage her adult son in this psychiatric condition with these vulnerabilities?

This patient and his family should be able to expect the provision of a reasonable consistency in diagnosis and treatment planning for co-occurring presentation, which includes precautions for safety and vulnerabilities. Predictably, what will follow is more covert THC abuse and more unpredictable and compulsive behavior with agitation and potential irrational combative behavior for patient B with direct unpredictable impact for his family. Lacking consistent medical team response to the urgency of patient B's comorbidity status, patient B and his family are even further removed from the

Guide to the Use of the Clinical Withdrawal Assessment Scale for Benzodiazepines

Person Report:

For each of the following items, circle the number that best describes how you feel.

Do you feel irritable?	0 Not at all	1	2	3	4 Very much so
Do you feel fatigued?	0 Not at all	1	2	3	4 Unable to function
Do you feel tense?	0 Not at all	1	2	3	4 Very much so
Do you have difficulties concentrating?	0 Not at all	1	2	3	4 Unable to concentrate
Do you have any loss of appetite?	0 Not at all	1	2	3	4 No appetite, unable to eat
Have you any numbness or burning on your face, hands or feet?	0 No numbness	1	2	3	4 Intense burning/numbness
Do you feel your heart racing? (palpitations)	0 No disturbance	1	2	3	4 Constant racing
Does your head feel full or achy?	0 Not at all	1	2	3	4 Severe headache

Fig. 4. Alcohol and other drug withdrawal: practice guidelines. Turning point alcohol and drug centre Inc. Clinical institute withdrawal assessment scale benzodiazepines. *Courtesy of* Turning Point Alcohol and Drug Centre, Inc., Victoria, Australia; with permission.

intervention they desperately need. Adult patient placement criteria for treatment of psychoactive substance use disorders are provided by the American Society of Addiction Medicine, and available via the American Society of Addiction Medicine **(Table 1)**.[48]

TREATMENT BARRIERS FOR CO-OCCURRING PSYCHIATRIC DISORDERS

Admission to critical care implies a critical incident resulting in need for intensive care. The critical incident can also be a psychiatric crisis. A psychiatric crisis requiring critical psychiatric care is usually identified by a threat of suicide or actual suicide attempt. Suicide attempts often include serious and life-threatening

Clinician Observations

Observe behaviour for sweating, restlessness and agitation		Observe tremor		Observe feel palms	
0	None, normal activity	0	No tremor	0	No sweating visible
1		1	Not visible, can be felt in fingers	1	Barely perceptible sweating, palms moist
2	Restless	2	Visible but mild	2	Palms and forehead moist, reports armpit sweating
3		3	Moderate with arms extended	3	Beads of sweat on forehead
4	Paces back and forth, unable to sit still	4	Severe, with arms not extended	4	Severe drenching sweats

Total Score Items 1 – 20

1–20 = mild withdrawal

41–60 = severe withdrawal

21–40 =moderate withdrawal

61–80 = very severe withdrawal

Fig. 5. (A) Alcohol and other drug withdrawal: practice guidlines. *Courtesy of* Turning Point Alcohol and Drug Centre, Inc., Victoria, Australia; with permission.

medical consequences, also requiring critical medical care. The patient admitted as a potential a danger to self or others, or because of a suicide attempt, may not have previously been assigned a psychiatric diagnosis. At this point a psychiatric referral is appropriate and usually initiated. There is not the discrepancy in assessment of priority of psychiatric care need in these kinds of critical care need presentations. It is uniformly agreed that suicide ideation or attempt are critical care level of need and justifiable reason for treatment intervention and hospital admission.

However, all patients admitted to critical care have experienced a critical incident resulting in a life disruption and often with extensive losses, or threat of loss. It has already been established that psychiatric referral and collaboration can reduce care requests, need for medication, and improve recovery.[32] A psychiatric assessment to determine degree of trauma experienced by the patient in critical care would affect improved recovery rates and prevention of extensive critical incident sequelae. This collaborative treatment approach, aligning psychiatry with primary treatment, is recommended by Centers for Substance Abuse treatment (CSAT).[23] According to CSAT, alignment of primary care with psychiatric care results in effective treatment, including "time sensitive screening, comprehensive assessment, specific clinical interventions of medications and psychological treatments."[23] This collaborative approach can result in resolution of patient and social system conflicts and positively impact the larger social system.

CRITICAL CARE TOOLS

Misuse of substances is invasive to the central nervous system (CNS). The most critical condition resulting from acute withdrawal is caused by CNS depressants (alcohol and benzodiazepines). When the blood concentration of CNS depressant precipitously drops, a condition termed acute withdrawal results.[49] A high blood concentration of CNS depressant (intoxication), immediately followed by acute withdrawal (precipitous drop in CNS depressant in level of blood concentration), can result in seizure and death. The medical intervention for acute withdrawal from CNS depressant is deliberate management of a controlled withdrawal of the same (CNS depressant), that is, benzodiazepines or phenobarbital to avoid seizure and death. Opioid, sedative, and hypnotic overdose can result in respiratory depression and also requires emergency response to ensure death does not occur from depression of respiration.[24]

Tools and scales are available to assist in determining degree of intoxication and level of withdrawal and provide evidence-based information aiding with decisions about medication management of acute withdrawal. These scales are available through the National Institutes of Health and include Addiction Research Foundation Clinical Institute Withdrawal Assessment of Alcohol (CIWA-Ar; **Fig. 1**),[50] Subjective Opiate Withdrawal Scale (SOWS; **Fig. 2**),[51] Objective Opiate Withdrawal Scale (OOWS; **Fig. 3**),[51] Stimulant Withdrawal Scale,[51] and Benzodiazepine Assessment Scale[52] (**Fig. 4**). (These scales are available on line by entering the name of the tool). Further discussion of management of substance abuse intoxication and withdrawal is found in the current literature.[2,24,49,50,53]

SUMMARY

Practicing within the paradigm of compartmentalized specially treatment without a collaborative practice is ineffective for the chemical dependency and dual diagnosis population. Chemical dependency is not well understood as a disease, evidenced by barriers cited from the 2005 Survey on Drug Use and Health.[15] Recovery from addiction and dual diagnosis logically demands an integrated and science-based treatment approach[47] with unified standards for care and improved educational standards for preparation of care providers (**Fig. 5**). Consultation and collaboration with addiction and psychiatric specialists is needed to establish consistency in standards for treatment and holistic care, essential for comorbidity. Continued learning and research about the complexity of the addiction process and comorbidity will provide continued accurate information about the harmful effects of alcoholism and drug abuse which in turn will empower individuals to make informed choices and result in better treatment and social policies.[37]

REFERENCES

1. Venes D. In: Taber's cyclopedic medical dictionary. 19th edition. Philadelphia: FA Davis; 2001.

2. Urschel HC. Healing the addicted brain. Naperville (IL): Source Books; 2009.
3. National Institute of Drug Abuse (NIDA). Drugs, brain, behavior: the science of addiction. Bethesda (MD): National Institute of Drug Abuse; 2007.
4. American Psychiatric Association. Diagnostic and statistical manual of mental disorders. 4th edition. Washington, DC: American Psychiatric Association Publishers; 2005.
5. Kalant H. Current state of knowledge about the mechanism of alcohol tolerance. Addict Biol 1998;22(1):67–76.
6. Kalant H. Research on tolerance: what can we learn from history?. Alcohol Clin Exp Res 1998;22:67.
7. Kalant H, LeBlanc A, Gibbons R. Tolerance to and dependency on, some non-opiate psychotropic drugs. Pharmacol Rev 1971;23:135.
8. Turner TB. Clinical aspects of ethanol tolerance and dependence. In: RHCJ Jr, editor. Clinical aspects of ethanol tolerance and dependence. Amsterdam: North Holland/Elsevier; 1980. p. 393.
9. Bush B, Shaw S, Cleary P, et al. Screening for alcohol abuse using the CAGE questionnaire. Am J Med 1987;82:231.
10. Searight HR. Screening for alcohol abuse in primary care: current status and research needs. Fam Pract Res J 1992;12:193.
11. Substance Abuse and Mental Health Services Administration (SAMHSA). Health effects of alcohol and other drugs on your body. Rockville (MD): U.S. Department of Health and Human Services; 2009.
12. Kaiser S. The importance of collaboration in the treatment of chemical dependency. Clin Nurse Specialist 2011;25:113.
13. Drug Abuse Warning Network (DAWN). Drug-related emergency department visits. Rockville (MD): Substance Abuse and Mental Health Services Administration; 2010.
14. Lichtenstein D, Spirito A, Zimmerman R. Assessing and treating co-occurring disorders in adolescents: examining typical practice of community-based mental health and substance use treatment providers. Commun Ment Health J 2010;46:252.
15. Substance Abuse and Mental Health Services Administration (SAMHSA). Results from the 2004 National Survey on Drug Use and Health: national findings. Rockville (MD): U.S. Department of Health and Human Services; 2005.
16. Substance Abuse and Mental Health Services Administration (SAMHSA). National Survey on Drug Use and Health. Bethesda (MD): National Institute of Drug Abuse; 2010.
17. Cychosz C. Alcohol and interpersonal violence: implications for educators. J Health Educ 1996;27(2):73–7.
18. McCollister K, French M, Fang H. The cost of crime to society: new crime specific estimates for policy and program evaluation. Drug Alcohol Depend 2010;108:98.
19. Office of National Drug Control Policy 2004. The economic costs of drug abuse in the United States 1992–2002. Washington, DC: Executive Office of the President; 2009.
20. Policy SIfH: Substance Abuse: The Nation's Number One Health Problem. In: Ericson N, editor. Schneider Institute for Health Policy, 2001, Brandeis University; 2004.
21. Kaiser S, Prendergast K. Nutritional links to substance abuse recovery. J Addict Nurs 2008;19:125.
22. Lisanti P. Assessment of the client for drug and alcohol use. Subst Abuse Educ Nurs 1991;15:151.
23. Substance Abuse and Mental Health Services Administration (SAMHSA). Report to Congress on the prevention and treatment of co-occurring substance abuse and mental health disorders in. Rockville (MD): U.S. Department of Health and Human Services; 2002.

24. Naegle MA, D'Avaonzo CE. Addictions and substance abuse. Upper Saddle River (NJ): Prentice Hall; 2001.
25. National Institute of Drug Abuse (NIDA). Comorbidity: addiction and other mental illnesses. In Volkow N, editor. Research Report Series. Bethesda (MD); National Institute of Drug Abuse; 2011.
26. U.S. Department of Health and Human Services, SAMHSA, CfMh, et al. Mental health: a report of the surgeon general. Rockville (MD):1999.
27. Drake RE, Mercer-McFadden C, Muser KT, et al. A review of integrated mental health and substance abuse treatment for patients with dual disorders. Schizophrenia Bull 1998;24:589–608.
28. Drake RE, McLaughlin P, Pepper B, et al. Dual diagnosis of major mental illness and substance disorder: an overview. San Francisco: Jossey-Bass; 1991.
29. Rand Corp. Office of National Drug Control Policy and the U.S. Army. Santa Monica (CA): Rand's Drug Policy Research Center; 1994.
30. Substance Abuse and Mental Health Services Administration (SAMHSA). Addictions treatment workforce development. Report to Congress. Broderick EBDM, Assistant Surgeon General, editor. Rockville (MD): U.S. Department of Health and Human Services; 2006.
31. Krupnick SLW. Navigating clinical care at the intersection of pain and addiction. MEDSURG Nursing 2009;18:381.
32. Harkness E, Bower P. On-site mental health workers delivering psychological therapy and psychosocial interventions to patients in primary care: effects on professional practice of primary care providers. Manchester (UK): National Primary Care Research and Development Center, University of Manchester; 2009.
33. Hart PD. The road to recovery: a landmark national study on public perceptions of alcoholism and barriers to treatment. Washington, DC: Rush Recovery Institute; 1998.
34. Volkow N. Comorbidity: addiction and other mental illnesses. NIDA News, September, 2011; p. 1–8.
35. Hoffman A, Heinemann ME. Substance abuse education in schools of nursing. J Nurs Educ 1987;26:282.
36. Kinney J, Price T, Bergen B. Impediments to alcohol education. J Stud Alcohol 1984;45:453.
37. Marcus M, Look D, Oswald L. Nursing care of clients with substance abuse in the hospital. St. Louis (MO): CV Mosby; 1995.
38. Church O. Curriculum for nursing education in alcohol and drug abuse. In: Fisk N, Neafsey P, editors. Storrs (CT): University of Connecticut; 1992.
39. Potter P, Perry A. Fundamentals of nursing. 3rd edition. St, Louis (MO): CV Mosby; 1993.
40. Kozier B, Erb G, Olivieri R. Fundamentals of nursing. Redwood City (CA): Addison-Wesley; 1991.
41. Scope and Standards of Addiction Nursing Practice American Nursing Association, International Nurses Society on Addiction. Washington, DC; 2004.
42. Savage SR, Horvath R. Opioid therapy of pain. In: Fiellin DA, Miller SC, Saitz R, editors. Principles of addiction medicine. 4th edition. Philadelphia: Lippincott Williams & Wilkins; 2009. p. 1329–51.
43. Carlson KK. Advanced critical care nursing. St. Louis (MO): Saunders-Elsevier; 2009.
44. International Society on Addiction Nursing. Scope and standards of addiction nursing practice. Washington, DC: American Nurses Association; 2008.
45. Craven M, Bland R. Better practices in collaborative mental health care: an analysis of the evidence base. Can J Psychiatry 2006;51:7S.

46. Murray RB, Zentner JP. Nursing assessment and health promotion strategies through the life span. Norwalk (CT): Appleton-Lange; 1993.
47. Kelly S, O'Grady K, Schwartz R, et al. The Community Assessment Inventory. Substance Abuse 2010;31:43.
48. Hoffman M, Halikas J, Mee-Lee D, et al. Patient placement criteria for the treatment of psychoactive substance use disorders. Washington, DC: American Society of Addiction Medicine; 1991.
49. Allen KM. Nursing care of the addicted client. Philadelphia: Lippincott; 1996.
50. Rousaville B, Tims F, Horton A, et al. Diagnostic source book on drug abuse research and treatment. Publication no. 93-3508. Rockville (MD): National Institutes of Health; 1993.
51. Handelsman L, Cochran KJ, Aronson MJ, et al. Two new rating scales for opiate withdrawal. Am J Drug Alcohol Abuse 1987;12:292–308.
52. Busto UE, Sykora K, Sellers EM. A clinical scale to assess benzodiazepine withdrawal. J Clin Psychopharmacol 1989;9(6):412–6.
53. National Institute of Drug Addiction. Principles of drug addiction treatment: a research-based guide. In: IUS Dept of Health and Human Services, editor. 2nd edition. Bethesda (MD): National Institute of Drug Addiction; 2009.

Survivors of Intimate Partner Violence: Implications for Nursing Care

Diane A. Hawley, PhD, RN, CCNS, CNE[a],*,
Alicia C. Hawley Barker, LMSW[b]

KEYWORDS

- Domestic violence • Health care • Abuse
- Intimate partner violence • Nursing
- Domestic violence screening • Spousal abuse

Ashley, a 26-year-old Caucasian woman, walked into the Emergency Department (ED) doubled over with abdominal pain. She also complained of a severe headache and nausea. Her husband of 2 years was present with her, attentive and concerned, helping her walk into the waiting room. The examination identified no medical concerns and she was discharged after 3 hours of observation. Her history included three ED visits in the past 3 years of similar presentation with the same conclusion of no medical diagnoses.

OVERVIEW

Violence against women by their husbands or intimate partners is one of the most common forms of violence. The fact that women rely on their abusers emotionally and economically brings complexity to the difficult situation. Domestic violence is an umbrella term that encompasses child, sibling, and elder abuse as well as intimate partner violence (IPV). Each form of abuse occurs within the confines of a domestic arrangement. The purpose of this article is to provide insight into the complexity of IPV in relation to acute care nursing as well as depict the psychological dynamics of IPV.

The terminologies of IPV versus domestic violence have been debated in the professional world for many years with regard to the type and scope of violence.[1] The

---

The authors have nothing to disclose.
[a] Harris College of Nursing and Health Sciences, Texas Christian University, TCU Box 298620, Fort Worth, TX 76129, USA
[b] Transitional Housing Coordinator, Hope's Door Inc. Domestic Violence Agency, 860 Avenue F Suite 100, Plano, TX 75074, USA
* Corresponding author.
E-mail address: d.hawley@tcu.edu

Crit Care Nurs Clin N Am 24 (2012) 27–39
doi:10.1016/j.ccell.2011.12.003
0899-5885/12/$ – see front matter © 2012 Elsevier Inc. All rights reserved.
ccnursing.theclinics.com

authors of this article define IPV as physical, sexual, or psychological harm by a current or former partner or spouse. The Centers for Disease Control (CDC) maintains that IPV is prevalent in both heterosexual and same-sex relationships. It is believed that the prevalence of IPV among lesbians, gay, bisexual, and transgender individuals is comparable to the domestic violence against heterosexual women.[1]

IPV can be represented by four categories to include physical violence, sexual violence, threats of physical or sexual violence, and psychological/emotional violence. Physical violence includes the "intentional use of physical force with the potential for causing death, disability, injury, or harm."[2(p11)] Leone Walker, author of *The Battered Woman*, categorized physical injuries based on various mechanisms and degrees of injury severity:

1. Serious bleeding injuries likely to need suturing
2. Internal injuries that lead to bleeding or organ failure
3. Skeletal damage of various sorts: ribs, vertebrae, skull, pelvic, jaw, arm and leg
4. Burns due to lit cigarettes, hot appliances, stove, iron, acid and scalding liquids.[3]

Sexual violence is multidimensional and includes offensive sexual contact or forcing an individual to engage in sexual acts.[2] Offensive sexual contact refers to actions of groping or grabbing a woman in a manner that is insulting. Forced sexual acts, whether completed or not, as well as refusing to practice safe sex, are forms of sexual violence. Sexual violence also involves an act or attempted act against someone who is unable to make an informed or conscious decision to engage in sexual activity whether due to illness, disability, or inability.[2] Statistics show that almost 7.8 million women have been raped by an intimate partner at some point in their lives.[1] Women under the influence of drugs or alcohol can be easy prey for sexual violence. Studies have found that stalking, forced sex, and physical abuse during a women's pregnancy are high-risk factors for female homicide.

Two forms of IPV that are less recognized in society include threats of violence as well as psychological or emotional abuse against an intimate partner. An example of a threat of violence is harming the family pet in lieu of the partner but saying "This is what will happen to you next." Psychological or emotional abuse can include "humiliating the victim, controlling what the victim can and cannot do, withholding information from the victim, deliberately doing something to make the victim feel diminished or embarrassed, isolating the victim from friends and family, and denying the victim access to money or other basic resources."[2(p13)] Not allowing the partner to drive and making her sit in the back seat of the car are both examples of psychological abuse. For many women, this type of abuse is far more harmful long term. Abusers may also tell their partners that they are ugly, worthless, and not good enough on a regular basis to emotionally abuse and diminish the survivor's self-esteem and self-worth.

Findings from the National Violence Against Women (NVAW) Survey, completed in 2000, revealed that roughly 1.5 million women and more than 800,000 men experience physical or sexual violence by intimate partners each year in the United States, although the findings may be underrepresented as it is believed that most violence is not reported to the police. This survey estimated that approximately one fifth of all rapes, one quarter of all physical assaults, and one half of all stalkings were believed to be reported to the police. The survey also found that women were much more likely to experience IPV than men.[4] According to the Bureau of Justice Statistics, 85% of domestic violence survivors are women.[5] Although the aforementioned NVAW survey revealed that men were also survivors of IPV, for the purposes of this article the authors focus on the majority of survivors who are women while recognizing that men experience IPV as well.

It is estimated that IPV costs the United States more than $5.8 billion annually, which is likely to be significantly underestimated because of medical care that is provided without screening for IPV. Studies show that 22% to 35% of women presenting to an ED who are treated for various injuries have experienced IPV.[6] The cost amount was gathered through analyzing medical and mental health care, lost productivity due to the violence, and a decrease in lifetime earnings.[1] By having a better understanding of the cost of IPV in the United States, society can have a more comprehensive picture of the impact of IPV within communities.

NATURE OF VIOLENCE

When discussing IPV, many individuals tend to use "victimization" terminology that often stems from the legal system. Instead of using the term "victim," the authors offer a strengths-based perspective that emphasizes resiliency by using the term "survivor." Much of society has a "victim blaming" mentality when questions arise about why a woman may choose to stay in an abusive relationship. One of the primary reasons women give for not disclosing the violence is shame. Society often blames a survivor for the abuse by saying she "asked for it" or "brought it on herself" because of characteristics such as the way she dresses or the way she does her hair and makeup. To use the term survivor instead of victim emphasizes her strength and ability to survive in the face of violence and adversity.

Rather than asking "Why does she stay in the relationship?" society might better ask "Why does he use violence?" There are numerous reasons why a woman might stay in an abusive relationship that are valid, and ultimately the decision is hers to make. She may stay because she loves the abuser; she may want to stay for the children; she may not have the financial means to support herself (and potentially the children) on her own; she may not have the support of friends and family; or she may not want to leave because of religious or cultural reasons.

IPV occurs on a continuum with regard to severity and frequency of violence. Some women may experience violence less frequently than others. IPV typically occurs in a cycle, however, that involves a tension-building phase that may include several heated arguments that ultimately build up to a violent episode. Many survivors describe the tension-building phase as "walking on eggshells." The violent episode can include anything from severe verbal criticism to a physically aggressive incident. After the violent episode, the survivor and abuser experience a honeymoon phase in which the abuser may apologize profusely, appear remorseful, shower her with gifts, and promise that he will never do it again. Each phase can last anywhere from one hour to one year depending on the relationship. When the honeymoon phase ends, the cycle starts over.

When working as nurses with survivors of IPV, it is important to understand the psychological impact surrounding the violence. IPV involves power and control. An abuser's belief that he is entitled to control another person is the basis for domestic violence. He believes violence is acceptable if it is necessary to get the desired outcome. The abuser uses various forms of violence as a means of exerting strength and authority over his partner. The Power and Control Wheel developed by the Domestic Abuse Intervention Project portrays the nature of power and control visually (**Fig. 1**). The key patterns of power and control include using intimidation, emotional or economic abuse, isolation, children, male privilege, coercion, threats, minimization, denial, and blaming.

Many domestic violence agencies and battering intervention programs utilize the Power and Control Wheel as a tool to educate both the survivors and abusers. Abuse toward an intimate partner is a conscious choice that an abuser makes. IPV is not

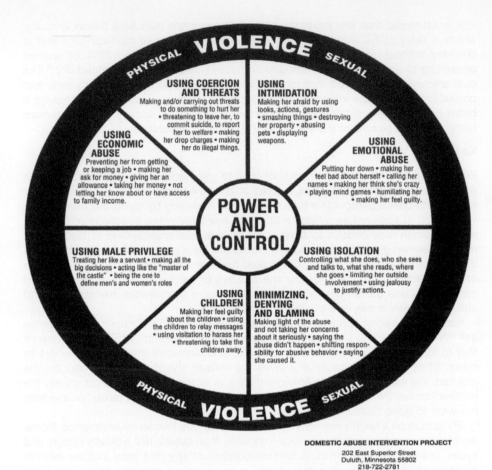

DOMESTIC ABUSE INTERVENTION PROJECT
202 East Superior Street
Duluth, Minnesota 55802
218-722-2781
www.duluth-model.org

Fig. 1. Power and Control Wheel illustrating the key patterns of power and control, including using intimidation, emotional or economic abuse, isolation, children, male privilege, coercion, threats, minimization, denial, and blaming. (*Courtesy of* Domestic Abuse Intervention Project, Duluth, MN; with permission.)

about anger. If the abuse was a true anger problem, then the abuser would be exerting power and control over, for example, the grocery store clerk, a co-worker, or a neighbor. Some individuals do need anger and aggression management counseling. IPV, however, is about a choice the abuser is making to be physically, sexually, or emotionally violent toward his partner.

Because survivors are often unaware of the tactics their abuser uses to gain power and domination, the use of the Power and Control Wheel can be an effective means of education. It is extremely common for survivors to be surprised by the many ways their abuser exerts control and power over them. Often they are shocked at the manipulation that has become the norm for them. It is crucial to educate survivors, nurses, and society about tactics of power and control in an abusive relationship as well as red flags to look for in abusers. By having a better understanding of the psychological aspects that violence has on the survivor, nurses can make informed decisions regarding screening and acute care, specifically relating to the survivor and family.

Two years later, Ashley, then 28 years old, presented with her husband to the same ED in severe respiratory distress, inspiratory stridor, vocal hoarseness, staccato speech, vaginal spotting, abdominal pain, and tenderness. She was 3 months pregnant with their first child. Ashley had some redness and significant edema to her neck. Her husband claimed she tripped on the living room rug and fell into the coffee table. Her respiratory rate was 38 breaths/min and SpO$_2$ was 88%. She was tachycardic, extremely frightened, and anxious about her pregnancy. Her hemoglobin level was 8.8 mg/dL and the sonogram could not rule out the possibility of placental separation. Ashley was sedated, intubated, placed on a ventilator, and admitted to the intensive care unit (ICU).

SCREENING

Virtually every American woman utilizes the health care system at some point in her life, whether it is for routine checkups, pregnancy, childbirth, illness, injury, or bringing her child in for health care. For millions of female survivors, the hospital can be a huge resource. The health care system currently has been successful in identifying and preventing significant public health problems. Just like routine screening for chronic health issues for early identification in all patients whether or not symptoms are apparent, this same approach to screening for IPV is appropriate. Nurses currently screen for common chronic conditions in which the prevalence is less than or similar to the IPV incidence. It is recommended that this routine screening for IPV take place in all primary care, urgent care, OB/Gyn and family planning, mental health, and inpatient settings.[7]

IPV brings millions of survivors to EDs and ICUs every year, and nurses often treat these women without inquiring about abuse or recognizing and addressing the cause of their underlying health problem, even if it is obvious. It is believed that 22% to 35% of all women presenting to an ED have symptoms of a problem related to partner abuse.[6] EDs and ICUs are the primary locations where people with injuries as a result of domestic violence enter the hospital environment. Only 2% to 8% of trauma patients are clinically recognized as abused.[8] It is known that survivors may have to be asked frequently about the presence of violence before they will acknowledge and seek assistance. Nurses must also know that if the woman does not acknowledge the abuse or refuses help, the survivor will still have likely listened carefully and it is not ever a failure on the nurse's part to question. There is research to suggest that women will disclose information about abuse more readily if health care professionals inquire.[9] Individuals who answer affirmatively about an incidence of violence can begin the process of helping themselves become free of violence in the future. Screening involves asking individuals about their personal experiences with being harmed. This questioning can be routine or based upon an index of suspicion. Routine, or sometimes referred to as universal screening, in the hospital environment means asking all persons aged 14 and older standard questions regarding domestic violence. Index of suspicion or incident-based screening relies on the supposed unusual clinical presentation or perceived demographic variables or risk factors that suggest a person is a survivor of violence.

Despite an enormous amount of research on female survivors of violence, there is no consensus of risk factors associated with IPV.[10] The lack of consistency in demographic and socioeconomic variables makes the Index of suspicion screening approach less than best practice for ED and ICU nurses specifically and hospital nurses generally. Because IPV impacts all socioeconomic statuses; religions; and

---

Box 1
Suggested screening questions

1. Framing Questions:

  a. Because violence is so common in many people's lives, I've begun to ask all my patients about it.

  b. I'm concerned that your symptoms may have been caused by someone hurting you.

  c. I don't know if this is a problem for you, but many of the women I see as patients are dealing with abusive relationships. Some are too afraid or uncomfortable to bring it up themselves, so I've started asking about it routinely.

  d. Some of the women and men we see here are hurt by their partners. Does your partner ever try to hurt you?

2. Direct Verbal Questions:

  a. Are you in a relationship with a person who physically hurts or threatens you?

  b. Did someone cause these injuries? Was it your partner/husband?

  c. Has your partner or ex-partner ever hit you or physically hurt you? Has he ever threatened to hurt you or someone close to you?

  d. Do you feel controlled or isolated by your partner?

  e. Do you ever feel afraid of your partner? Do you feel you are in danger? Is it safe for you to go home?

  f. Has your partner ever forced you to have sex when you didn't want to? Has your partner ever refused to practice safe sex?

Produced by Futures Without Violence, 100 Montgomery Street, The Presidio San Francisco, CA 94129-1718. (415) 678-5500 TTY:(800) 595-4889. Available at: www.futureswithoutviolence.org; Used with permission.

---

racial, cultural and ethnic groups, it is difficult to pinpoint a specific profile of a survivor. It is known that poverty and lack of education are considered risk factors, although some believe that the more educated and wealthy a woman is, the more possible it is for her to circumvent the health care setting when help is needed. Culture and religious affiliations, along with language barriers, impact health care–seeking behaviors and possibly the identification of survivors of violence. Different cultures define what constitutes domestic violence in ways unique to the American perspective. The vagueness of a survivor profile is the very reason why screening should be conducted on all women, both adults and adolescents seeking medical attention in a hospital environment.

Routine screening has been recommended by many organizations interested in the welfare of women in the United States.[11] Screening is only as effective as the tool used to identify the survivor. There is ample evidence acknowledging simple direct questioning as the most valuable means of facilitating disclosure of IPV and thus discovering a case. **Box 1** has suggestions for framing the context and asking questions in identifying IPV situations. There seems to be conflicting research as to whether routines to questioning have been shown to increase detection rates. Several studies suggest that screening practices have not been effective in identifying survivors of IPV. On the other hand, one can find quality studies that have shown increased screening resulting in increased detection.[12]

A huge, confounding variable to routine screening is the fact that there seems to be insufficient research to link routine screening to better intervention strategies or improved outcomes for survivors.[13] There is much difficulty in designing longitudinal research studies to measure the impact of detection on such things as accessing services, initiating safety plans, or reducing mortality rates. One issue could be a lack of a comprehensive approach to the treatment of IPV in health care facilities where a case is identified. An argument could be made questioning the value of routine screening if there are insufficient processes in place to address the abuse. Also, inadequate interventions can lead to psychological stress, increased tension with possible escalation of abuse, loss of home residence or financial resources, deterioration of the family structure, loss of autonomy, and even lost work hours.

There seem to be some overarching reasons why nurses have difficulty in routinely asking patients questions regarding potential violence. Having inadequate knowledge and skills about IPV is certainly one cause for struggling or choosing not to ask questions of all women. It is known that educational programs do not increase detection rates of abuse. Nurses sometimes feel that the screening questions are inappropriate for the type of presentation the woman is exhibiting. The American Nurses Association[14] and the American Association of Colleges of Nursing[15] both have position statements recommending that all professional nurses have domestic violence content and clinical experiences within their nursing education programs. Still, there continues to be a lack of violence-related content and planned clinical learning experiences within a majority of accredited nursing programs.

A second explanation for difficulties in routine screening is related to insufficient institutional resources such as privacy areas or after-hour services when many cases of IPV present to the hospital. There also could be a lack of cues or prompts in an assessment or history document to remind nurses to ask appropriate questions. Another concern is that if the nurse pursues the issue of violence with the survivor, other problems might be exposed that he or she as a nurse might not have time to deal with.

The attitude of nurses has an impact on routine screening. Some nurses might be naïve about the prevalence and complex nature of abuse and assume that it is not an issue for the population they serve. Another premise could be that some nurses believe that IPV is a private matter and fear that patients would be upset or offended if asked about violence or that the line of questioning may lead to a breakup of the family. Nurses may lack the empathy, understanding, or respect to care for these patients. Avoidance might play a part in encounters with survivors because they might be dealing with abuse in their own personal lives. Two studies indicated that 27% to 31% of nurses reported personal experiences with IPV.[16,17] These findings support the statistic that one in four women experiences abuse by an intimate partner.[6] Nurses who are or have experienced personal violence may have difficulty providing appropriate care to survivors of violence. Finally, the nurse may feel the need to concentrate on his or her comfort area, which may likely be focusing on physical needs rather than the true underlying mental health problem for the survivor.

Patients generally find being asked about violence acceptable and support routine screening. Olive found that survivors felt that they would also have liked to have been asked about family life and emotional abuse as well when questioned.[11] A worthwhile stance for IPV is to consider any intervention that seeks to reduce the incidence of presentations within hospitals as valuable.

INTERVIEWING

It must be said that women in abusive relationships rarely volunteer information about abuse to health care providers. Everything that can be done to help the individual feel safe and comfortable with nurses and the environment needs to be encouraged. Nurses need exceptional interviewing and observational skills when caring for these survivors and all involved parties.

A desirable setting is critical for the interview process. Total privacy is a must. One way to assist in creating this privacy is to post in all waiting rooms a policy of guaranteeing all patients a private interview on admission. If children older than the age of 2 are accompanying the survivor, ask another staff or family member to stay with them. It is imperative that no exceptions be made to this rule no matter how emphatic, charming, or attentive a partner can be. A second attempt at requesting the partner to leave the room is necessary if the partner is reluctant or belligerent. Solicit the help of a coworker to make an excuse to speak with him, such as needing further contact information. If these attempts fail, discontinue efforts because this could trigger an escalation of violence by the abuser. Excuses of staying in the room to interpret for the patient cannot be a reason, so it is important to consult a professional interpreter when necessary, preferably of the same sex and cultural background as the patient. Be sure to remember that same-sex partners can be abusers as well.

The interview should begin by sitting down next to your patient. Sitting will suggest that you are not rushed and are interested in spending time with her. Your nonverbal behavior needs to be in check and show caring and empathy. Arms or legs crossed certainly suggest closed and uninterested posturing. Facial expressions can also reflect both genuine sincerity and hurried thoughts.

Begin a conversation with a reassurance that what she tells you will be confidential but also inform her of the limits of that confidentiality. Be aware that there are usually limits to confidentiality such as any child abuse or neglect, elder abuse or neglect, abuse to a person with a disability, sexual abuse by a mental health provider, if the medical records are subpoenaed by court or if the patient is threatening to harm herself or others. A few states have laws mandating reporting of IPV. Research has been conducted regarding mandatory reporting of IPV and some of the barriers that might inhibit reporting. They include reasons such as not having enough evidence, survivors not wanting the episode recorded, nurse/patient confidentiality, disrupting family relationships, fear of retaliation, being uncomfortable with the situation, problem not serious enough, and many more.[10]

It is important early on in an interview with a survivor to acknowledge that abuse is common in our society and make a hopefully true disclaimer that all patients are asked questions about whether they are in a harmful relationship and whether they feel safe. Nurses should be alert to clues in a woman's behavior, patterns of physical injuries and illnesses, and the behavior of the patient's partner. Behaviors that raise suspicion are delaying the seeking of treatment for an injury or appearing embarrassed, anxious, evasive, or depressed. Some survivors talk of harming themselves. They may have enough comfort with you to express fear about returning home or fear for the children. Often there is a history of frequent emergency or office visits for injuries. Another typical behavior is to make excuses for her abuser such as saying he has a psychiatric history or problems with alcohol or drugs.

One should suspect IPV when there are unexplained bruises, lacerations, burns, fractures, or multiple injuries in various stages of healing, especially in areas normally covered with clothing. Occasionally injuries not reported by the survivor are discovered and in need of medical attention, such as neck markings suggestive of strangulation when the primary presentation might be a fracture. A usual presentation is a woman not appropriately dressed for the weather, such as wearing long sleeves in the summer because someone has grabbed her arm with such force it caused significant fingerprint bruise markings. Often these injuries and illnesses do not reflect the nature of the presentation to the hospital. The partner's behavior can be either very kind or very hostile. The partner could be uncooperative, forceful, reluctant to leave, domineering, and insist on speaking for the survivor or could appear to be very attentive, loving, charismatic, and genuine toward the survivor.

Noting behavioral cues is a much greater challenge in the intensive care setting when the woman is being treated for a serious enough condition that communication is hindered because of unconsciousness or intubation. In this instance, an abuser will speak for the patient and will not want to leave the woman's bedside. This might be perceived by a critical care nurse as thoughtful vigilance if IPV is not considered. One action on the part of the abuser that might tip the nurse off to violence is the insistence on knowing the precise means of verbal, written, or gesture communication the patient had in his absence.

Critically ill patients who are able to communicate by some means and stable enough to interview should be asked the usual routine questions of history, especially related to feeling safe at home and social relationships with a partner that can lead to harm. As mentioned previously, any interviewing of an ICU survivor needs to be done in a private and safe environment. When abuse is suspected but the woman claims an unusual accounting or is silent, the nurse should continue to pursue the issue with a nonjudgmental demeanor. Nurses must realize that many women hesitate to disclose this devastating information until they can feel comfortable that the nurse wants to hear the specifics or they can handle the details. One can imagine instances in which the nurse's interview leads to an immediate shutdown of discussion about the abuse versus another interview with much elaboration of an abusive relationship, all related to the nurse either pursuing with genuine interest or dropping the discussion prematurely.

It is important the nurse respond to any disclosure of abuse in an appropriate and genuine manner. If there is a negative response by the nurse such as doubt, disinterest, or discounting the explanation of abuse, it can be assumed that the survivor will attempt to avoid health care services in the future. The nurse must avoid using words or phrases that suggest minimization or fault such as just, only, why, and you should. One question that often implies blame is "Why don't you just leave him?" A positive response of concern, support, and referrals would result in hope for the survivor and her options.

A mistake the nurse must not make is to criticize the woman's abuser. Human nature will err on the side of defending her partner's redeeming qualities rather than acknowledge the problematic or abusive action. After all, in her mind there must have been an attraction to the man that she is still holding on to. It cannot be assumed that the woman wants to end the relationship at this time either. Many times the survivor is still in love with the abuser and depends on him for economic and emotional support. Usually no protective order or police officer can protect the woman from harm and there is the potential for an investigation to portray the survivor as an unfit parent and possibly take the children away. Survivors know that leaving can be more dangerous than staying. Fear often plays a part in remaining in the relationship. Survivors understand the very real statistic that of victims killed by their abusers, 70% were trying to leave.[18] A survivor knows her own situation and understands the consequences of her actions. It is important to note that the nurse is not a rescuer in this instance nor should he or she attempt to counsel the survivor to prosecute her partner. The nurse has a responsibility to make sure the survivor is making her decisions with accurate information and with a network of support.

INTERVENTIONS

Nursing care begins with triaging the patient's physiologic care needs and stabilizing the patient. Women who are under anesthesia, intubated, unconscious, or sedated may not be able to communicate or to comprehend the situation at hand. A medical response to the abuse could be ignored or stalled because of short hospital stays and transfers to other areas. The lack of continuity can hinder addressing the abuse as health care providers. The key will be to alert and involve a liaison person who can follow the patient through the hospital stay and even after discharge into the community. Collaborating with the survivor's primary care provider, a case manager, or social worker will be imperative for that patient's future.

It is essential for the nurse to realize the importance of accurately reflecting clinical findings in the medical record. IPV is a crime, and as such, in a court of law, medical record entries can determine a case. To protect your patient's confidentiality, never place her chart on a counter or anywhere else visible. Be sure any computer monitor is turned off. Be sure that she knows that her medical records are available if she needs them for legal purposes. How the hospital visit is documented can decide whether there is justice for the abused.

It is important to use terminology carefully or the nurse will lose credibility in the court of law. Wound terms can be misused or inappropriate for the situation. For example, ecchymosis is a hemorrhagic spot on the skin or mucous membrane usually secondary to an underlying pathology such as thrombocytopenia. Trauma does not cause ecchymosis. A likely better term would be contusion or bruise to accurately reflect the injury. The injuries/wounds need to be described in a narrative based on appearance, color, and size. It is not recommended to suggest an estimated age for bruising based on color. There are wounds that are defensive in nature when the survivor attempts to protect herself from the assailant. Cuts or injuries on the upper extremities, especially an ulnar fracture of the arm without a radial fracture, are suggestive of abuse. When the back, buttocks, or occipital areas have injuries it could be the individual had curled into a ball to protect herself.

Documentation needs to be particularly attentive to accuracy, detail, and objectivity. One important documentation suggestion is to diagram injuries on a body map and ask for consent to photograph and take pictures as appropriate. If the violence occurred that same day, it might be appropriate to talk with the survivor about follow-up pictures in a few days once the bruising has fully developed, either while she is in the hospital or at the police station.

It is imperative that all written narratives, diagram mappings, and pictures be congruent and support each other's description of the injuries. Many signs of IPV can be noted without ever asking a question or getting a response. Cowering to any touch or not making eye contact are two examples of nonverbal cues of concern. Record the demeanor and actions of both the survivor and the partner. Be sure to narrative write who the suspected abuser is. Specifically write the relationship of the abuser to the patient. Note as much information about the abuser as possible to include all identifying information such as address and date of birth. Use direct quotes as much as possible, even with the possibility of slang or foul language, and place them in quotation marks. Do not paraphrase language in an attempt to enter into the record a professional accounting. Unsavory language if used will convey the context of the scene. A paraphrasing of statements rather than the verbatim words will lose credibility in a court of law. It is important to record the patient's and partner's exact words accurately. Do not use the word "alleged" in the belief that you might be wrongfully accusing. This word will imply that you as the nurse have concerns about the truth in the survivor's story. Also be extremely careful when you use words such as "refused" or "uncooperative" to describe the survivor, as they are subjective, negative comments to things that may be or have been out of her control. Entering statements in quotations helps the nurse maintain neutrality. On the other hand, do not enter into the medical record survivor statements that are not important to medical care such as "I'm not a good wife." These could be damaging to the survivor in legal proceedings. As discussed earlier, a harmful effect of abuse is a demoralized sense of self for abused women. Nurses need to repeat often that the abuse is not their fault. Talking about the violence validates the significance of the problem for the abused. Often praise the survivor for her strength and courage. Be sure that you are documenting the education you did with her and any resources you gave her to include referrals to social services.

SAFETY

In instances in which IPV is known or disclosed, the most immediate safety need is to determine where the abuser is at the time the survivor is seeking medical attention. It is also important to know whether children were witnesses to the abuse that took place and if they were harmed. If the abuse involved children, it is paramount that you find out if they are in a safe environment now. You may not have any choice but to contact law enforcement and Child Protective Services because child abuse is a mandatory reportable offense. The survivor needs to be asked whether she would like to file a report with law enforcement if not already involved.

It is important to assess whether there might be a coexisting mental health problem such as severe depression, suicidal ideations, or drug/alcohol abuse that would lead to an unsafe situation for the survivor or abuser. Any of these circumstances would require further evaluation by a mental health specialist. The survivor needs to be asked about any threats of homicide, suicide, or access to a gun. The key to safety beyond the immediate needs is related to the survivor understanding the level of risk she is experiencing. Only the survivor can know when it is time to leave. The average survivor leaves her abuser seven times before she is successful.[18] If the woman decides to remain in the relationship, safety considerations need to be discussed. The survivor may not be interested in discussing this, so you might use a framing statement such as "Let's talk about ways to help you and your children stay safe." The nurse should inquire about the worst incidence of violence to date to help the survivor understand her level of risk and whether there is an escalation to the violence. It is important to identify a safe place for the children and her if the abuse escalates out of control. Having a code phrase that a friend/neighbor knows when help is needed is another safety strategy. An example of a code phrase might be "Did you talk with Dr. Jones today?" In the event that a survivor uses a code phrase with her contact, that individual knows the action(s) to take such as calling 9-1-1 on behalf of the survivor.

Some additional tips include keeping important papers, cash, credit cards, spare clothes, important phone numbers, as well as medications for the survivor and any children in a safe place. It is also important to suggest always leaving shoes, purse, cell phone, and keys near the front door and plan an escape route if she might need to leave the house quickly. It is imperative that the survivor know that she must not hesitate to call the police if there are any instinctive feelings or hints of danger.

The discharge plan for this survivor includes giving her referral information. Resources need to be offered, such as a 24-hour emergency hotline, domestic violence agency websites, names and numbers responsive to IPV, housing or shelter resources, area support groups, and legal counsel information. Remember to be sensitive to the fact that these women might very well not want to bring any written literature home with them for fear of their abuser discovering the documents. A suggestion is to write down only phone numbers on a prescription slip or discharge form for the woman to keep in her wallet.

SUMMARY

As IPV increases in our society, hospitals need to prepare to best meet the needs of these individuals. Hospitals should have policies that encourage critical care nurses to consider abuse with the patients they serve. These policies need to ensure private, confidential interviewing of all patients and standardize the follow-up for any identified cases. There needs to be routine prompts in an assessment and history that clarify whether the person is in a violent situation. Nurses should understand more specifically the context of IPV and know the community resources available to survivors of this violence. Last, nurses need to recognize the physical, psychological, and emotional support they can give to these individuals. The acronym RADAR, developed by the Massachusetts Medical Society, succinctly represents the thought processes that need to occur with all domestic violence cases[6]:

R: Perform *routine* screening.

A: *Ask* direct questions.

D: *Document* findings.

A: *Assess* patient (and children) safety.

R: *Review* patient options and provide *referrals.*

The ultimate aim for hospitals is to empower nurses to provide compassionate care for survivors and establish emotional climates conducive to IPV disclosure and subsequent care.

REFERENCES

1. National Center for Injury Prevention and Control. Costs of intimate partner violence against women in the United States. Atlanta (GA): Centers for Disease Control and Prevention; 2003.
2. Saltzman LE, Fanslow JL, McMahon P, et al. Intimate partner violence surveillance: uniform definitions and recommended data elements, version 1.0. Atlanta (GA): Centers for Disease Control and Prevention, National Center for Injury Prevention and Control; 2002.
3. Walker Z. The battered women. New York: Harper and Row; 1979.
4. Tjaden P, Thoennes N. Extent, nature, and consequences of intimate partner violence: findings from the National Violence Against Women Survey. Washington, DC: U.S. Department of Justice; 2000. Publication No. NCJ 181867. Available from: www.ojp.usdoj.gov/nij/pubs-sum/181867.htm. Accessed October 30, 2011.
5. Bureau of Justice Statistics Crime Data Brief, Intimate Partner Violence, 1993–2001. February 2003. Washington, DC: Bureau of Justice Statistics.
6. Fulton D. Recognition and documentation of domestic violence in the clinical setting. Crit Care Nurs 2000;23(2):26–34.
7. Family Violence Prevention Fund. Preventing domestic violence: clinical guidelines on routine screening. Futures without Violence. San Francisco (CA): Family Violence Prevention Fund; 1999. p. 1–23.

8. Thurston E, Tutty L, Eisener E, et al. Domestic violence screening rates in a community health center urgent care clinic. Res Nurs Health 2007;30:611–9.
9. Hegarty K, Taft A. Overcoming the barriers to disclosure and inquiry of partner abuse for women attending general practice. Austral New Zeal J Public Health 2001;25(5): 433–7.
10. Amar A, Cox C. Intimate partner violence: implications for critical care nursing. Crit Care Nurs Clin North Am 2006;18:287–96.
11. Olive P. Care for emergency department patients who have experienced domestic violence: a review of the evidence base. J Clin Nurs 2007;16:1736–48.
12. Smith J, Rainey S, Smith K, et al. Barriers to the mandatory reporting of domestic violence encountered by nursing professionals. J Trauma Nurs 2008;15(1):9–16.
13. Ramsey J, Richardson J, et al. Should health professionals screen women for domestic violence? Systematic review. Br Med J 2002;325;314–27.
14. American Nurses Association. Position statement: physical violence against women. 2000. Available at: http://nursingworld.org. Accessed October 30, 2011.
15. American Association of Colleges of Nursing. Violence as a public health problem. Available at: http://www.aach.nche.edu/Pulbications/positions/violence.htm. Accessed October 30, 2011.
16. Ellis J. Barriers to effective screening for domestic violence by registered nurses in the emergency department. Crit Care Nurs Q 1999;22(1):27–41.
17. Moore M, Zaccaro D, Parsons L. Attitudes and practices of registered nurses toward women who have experienced domestic violence. JOGNN 1998;27:175–82.
18. Berlinger J. Taking an intimate look at domestic violence. Nursing 2004;34(10):42–6.

Assessment of Risk for In-Hospital Suicide and Aggression in High-Dependency Care Environments

Leslie Rittenmeyer, RN, PsyD, CNS, CNE

KEYWORDS

- In-hospital suicide • Aggression
- High-dependency environments • Staff training

The primary concern in any clinical setting is patient safety. Owing to variability in the characteristics of the patient population, the critical care environment presents its own unique set of safety challenges. This article addresses two of those: risk of in-hospital (outside the psychiatric unit) suicide and potential for family or patient aggression.

CRITICAL CARE ENVIRONMENT

Stress in the critical care environment has been widely reported.[1-4] For most patients and their significant others, admission to a high-dependency unit constitutes a crisis. Crisis often occurs when a series of events happen that creates a situation that is perceived as threatening. The physiological, emotional, and behavioral responses to these feelings will vary from person to person because aside from their personal property, all patients bring with them their own unique coping abilities, strengths, constraints, and preexisting mental and physical conditions. This is exactly why there is potential for incidences of both suicide and aggression in this environment. If people's behavior were always predictable, how they might respond to a particular situation would not be such a concern.

The complexity of intervening on many different levels is demanding for critical care nurses and the reason why job stress is common. In addition to caring for patients and their significant others, nurses must cope with high mortality rates, ethical dilemmas, end-of-life decisions, the interdisciplinary team, conflicting value disputes, and an enormous workload. It is especially because of this that nurses in this setting must be

The author has nothing to disclose.
School of Nursing, Purdue University Calumet, 220 169th Street, Hammond, IN 46323, USA
E-mail address: rittenme@purduecal.edu

Crit Care Nurs Clin N Am 24 (2012) 41–51
doi:10.1016/j.ccell.2012.01.002
0899-5885/12/$ – see front matter © 2012 Elsevier Inc. All rights reserved.

particularly attuned to changes in patient behavior that might signal distress. Early detection and intervention are key in keeping patients safe.

RISK FOR SUICIDE

Whereas psychiatric units are designed (or should be) for suicide prevention, this is not always the case with other areas in the general hospital. In one study it was found that even psychiatric units are not always designed with safety in mind.[5,6] Some environmental risk factors include anchor points for hanging, potentially dangerous materials that can be used for self harm, and problems encountered in trying to make any environment completely safe.[5,6] Methods of self-harm that are commonly used in health care environments include hanging, jumping, cutting with a sharp object, drug overdose, and strangulation.[5,6] There are some specific means for self-harm in the general hospital setting that have been used to complete a suicide: bell cords, bandages, tubing, sheets, and restraint belts.[7] System constraints create risk as well, for example, poor assessment, observation, and intervention; insufficient staff training; inadequate staffing; poor communication; and lack of information about suicide prevention and referral sources.[5,8]

IN-HOSPITAL SUICIDE OUTSIDE BEHAVIORAL HEALTH AND PSYCHIATRIC UNITS

Patient suicide or attempted suicide resulting in serious disability while a patient is being cared for in a health care facility is one of the National Quality Forum's (NQF) Health Care "never events." The term "never event" was first introduced in 2001 by Ken Kizer, MD, former CEO of the NQF, in reference to particularly shocking medical errors (such as wrong-site surgery) that should never occur.[9] The Joint Commission (TJC) labels in-hospital suicide a sentinel event.[10] A sentinel event is an unexpected occurrence involving death or serious physical or psychological injury, or the risk thereof. In 1998, TJC issued a Sentinel Event Alert on preventing inpatient suicides with a focus on general hospitals and prevention of suicide in medical/surgical arenas and emergency departments.[11] This report was updated in 2010.[5] A goal of the 2010 report was to provide information that would ensure that patients outside of the psychiatric unit are appropriately screened and cared for. They note in the report that:

> While psychiatric setting are designed to be safe for suicidal individuals and have staff with specialized training, typically, medical /surgical units and emergency departments are not designed or assessed for suicide risk and do not have staff that have specialized training to deal with suicidal individuals. Not surprisingly, suicidal individuals often are admitted to general hospitals immediately following suicide attempts or they seek help in hospital emergency departments – often at the urging of family or friends – when they are most desperate, these patients are known " at risk" for suicide.[5(p1)]

Many patients who kill themselves in general hospital inpatient units within the general hospital have no psychiatric history or history of previous suicide attempt. They are not known to be at risk for suicide.[7] TJC reports that suicide has been ranked in the top five most frequently reported sentinel events since 1995. The Sentinel Event Database includes 827 reports of inpatient suicides. Of the 827 reports:

- 14.25% occurred in the nonbehavioral health units of general hospitals (eg, medical or surgical units, intensive care unit [ICU] oncology, telemetry).
- 8.02% occurred in the emergency department of general hospitals.

Box 1
Risk factors for suicide

- Suicidal ideation
- Suicidal behavior
- Psychiatric diagnosis
- Family history of suicide attempt or psychiatric illness
- Physical health problems
- Traumatic brain injuries, posttraumatic stress disorder
- Delirium or dementia
- Chronic pain or intense acute pain

- Poor prognosis or prospect of certain death
- Social stressors such as financial strain, unemployment
- Relational problems, divorce
- Substance abuse
- Hopelessness
- Disability

Data from The Joint Commission. A follow-up report on preventing suicide: focus on medical surgical/nursing and the emergency department. Sentinel event alert 2010; Issue 46. Available at: http://www.jointcommission.org/SentinelEvents/; and Tischler C, Reiss N. Inpatient suicide: preventing a common sentinel event. Gen Hosp Psychatiry 2009;31:103–9.

- 2.45% occurred in other nonpsychiatric settings (eg, home care, critical access hospitals, long-term care hospitals, and physical rehabilitation hospitals).[5]

SUICIDE ASSESSMENT
Who Is At Risk?

Physical illness and mental disorders have been recognized as risk factors for suicide.[12] Patients who have a physical illness are two to three times more likely to complete a suicide than those who do not.[13,14] Annually, approximately 650,000 individuals require emergency room treatment in U.S. medical centers as the result of attempted suicide.[15] Identified risk factors for suicide are listed in **Box 1**.

Warning Signs

There are numerous warning signs distinct from the risk factors that are associated with the increased feelings of desperation and can represent imminent risk.[5] A summary of these signs is provided in **Box 2**.

Box 2
Suicidal warning signs

- Irritability
- Increased anxiety
- Agitation
- Impulsivity
- Decrease emotional reactivity
- Complaining of unrelenting pain
- Refusal to see visitors

- Refusing medications
- Requesting early discharge
- Meeting the diagnostic criteria for depression
- Feelings of worthlessness
- Decreased interest in treatment of prognosis
- Refusing to eat

Data from The Joint Commission. A follow-up report on preventing suicide: Focus on medical surgical/nursing and the emergency department. Sentinel event alert 2010; Issue 46. Available at: http://www.jointcommission.org/SentinelEvents/; Bostwick J, Rackley S. Completed suicide in medical/surgical patients: who is at risk? Curr Psychiatry Rep 2007;9:242–6; and Wint D, Akil M. Suicidality in the general hospitalized patient. Hosp Physician 2006; January:13–8.

> **Box 3**
> **Stages of crisis development**
> - The individual or family is in a state of homeostasis.
> - A stressful event or events occur.
> - The event is perceived as a threat.
> - Well known coping skills are applied but fail to reduce the threat.
> - A period of disequilibrium occurs with a decrease of problem-solving ability and increase in feelings of anxiety and depression.
> - The problem is either resolved or personal disintegration occurs.

Suicide assessment should become part of nurses' daily assessment routine. Accordingly, nurses must keep the suicide risk factors and warning signs in their conscious mind, as they do other assessment criteria. A clinical story illustrates this. There was a tragic incident in which a male patient was admitted to an intensive care unit after an uncompleted suicide attempt with carbon monoxide. Even though his admission was the result of a suicide attempt, the staff failed to assess him for his level of suicidality. He had been on unit before and was labeled a "frequent flyer." He died in the ICU by hanging himself with his belt from the intravenous medication pole. In conducting an autopsy on the circumstances of this incident it was found that besides having a previous and recent suicide attempt, he also had a history of 12 of the risk factors listed in **Box 1**. Ask yourself the following questions: What could have been done to prevent this? Was it preventable? What do you think a reasonable and prudent nurse would have done? How would you have responded?

In addition to being cognizant of the suicide risk factors it is also important to be cognizant of the warning signs as distinct from the risk factors because some patients will not have many or any of the risk factors but will display suicide warning signs. Nurses must always keep in mind that given the right circumstances any person's coping abilities can become overwhelmed. The stages of crisis development provide a picture of how this might happen (**Box 3**).

More specifically to this point, in a study that looked at the characteristics of medical/surgical patients who died by suicide found that:

- There appeared to be an impulsive nature to these suicides.
- Few had known histories of psychiatric illness or suicidal behavior.
- Some were judged—after the fact—to have been agitated while experiencing an undiagnosed depression or delirium at the time of their deaths.
- Some were distraught by an emotional rift.
- Almost none of the deaths involved lengthy planning.
- Most used means readily at their disposal such as stairwells, window curtain rods, and bathroom fixtures.
- Staff sometimes unwittingly provided the instrument of death in the form of medical equipment.[7(p245)]

INTERVENTION/PREVENTION

The difficulty of ensuring patient safety in the critical care arena is due in part to the fact that there are a myriad of different types of patients that need high-dependency care. Suicide prevention is aimed at the individual needs of the patient. For instance, if the patient is admitted with a psychiatric diagnosis or a suicide attempt one would look to the patient's psychiatric history for guidance. This approach might not be helpful for other types of patients. "Medical/Surgical patients may be less likely than psychiatric patients to display traditional risk factor such as substance abuse. They are much more likely to have agitation propelled by delirium induced by a medical/surgical condition."[7(p245)]

The Practice Recommendations from the Registered Nurses' Association of Ontario (RNAO) assessment and care of adults at risk for suicidal ideation and behavior clinical guideline provides guidance for assessing and caring for adults at risk for suicidal ideation and behavior.[16]

The guideline has the following objectives:

1. To assist nurses working in diverse practice settings to provide evidence-based care to adults at risk for suicidal ideation and behaviors
2. To provide nurses with recommendations, based on the best available evidence, related to the assessment and management of adults at risk for suicidal ideation and behavior
3. To increase nurses' comfort, confidence, and competence in this practice area, in order to enhance safety for their clients and to lower the impact of suicide for society
4. To provide support to the nurse in her or his care of the suicidal patient

The following evidence-based practice recommendations are meant to support nurses' clinical decision making, without implying that they hold more weight than one's clinical expertise and judgment in any clinical situation.[16]

1. The nurse will take seriously all statements made by the client that indicates, directly or indirectly, a wish to die by suicide, and all available information that indicates a risk for suicide.
2. The nurse works toward establishing a therapeutic relationship with clients at risk for suicidal ideation and behavior.
3. The nurse works with the client to minimize the feelings of shame, guilt, and stigma that may be associated with suicidality, mental illness, and addiction.
4. The nurse provides care in keeping with the principles of cultural safety/cultural competence.
5. The nurse assesses and manages factors that may impact the physical safety of both the client and the interdisciplinary team.
6. The nurse assesses for protective factors associated with suicide prevention.
7. The nurse obtains collateral information from all available sources: family/friends/community support/medical records and medical health professionals.
8. The nurse mobilizes resources based on the client's assessed level of suicide risk–associated needs.
9. The nurse ensures that observation and therapeutic engagement reflect the client's changing suicide risk.
10. The nurse uses a mutual problem-solving approach to facilitate the client's understanding of how he or she perceives his or her own problems and generate solutions.
11. The nurse fosters hope with the suicidal client.
12. The nurse is aware of current treatments to provide advocacy, referral, monitoring, and health teaching interventions, as appropriate.
13. The nurse identifies persons affected by suicide that may benefit from resources and supports and refers as appropriate.

14. Nurse may initiate and participate in a debriefing process with other team members regarding organizational protocol.
15. The nurse seeks support for clinical supervision when working with adults at risk for suicidal ideation and behavior to become aware of the emotional impact of the nurse and enhance clinical practice.
16. Nursing curricula should corporate content on mental health issues, including suicide risk reduction and prevention, in a systematic manner to promote core competencies and mental health practice.
17. Health care organizations that admit suicidal clients must provide a safe physical environment that minimizes access to the means for self-injurious behavior.
18. In health care organizations that admit suicidal patients, nursing staff complements should be appropriate to the patient/nurse ratio and to the staff mix to safely meet the unpredictable needs of acutely suicidal patients.
19. Organizations ensure the critical incidents involving suicidal behavior are reviewed systematically to identify opportunities for learning at all levels of service delivery.
20. Organizations develop policies and structures related to peer debriefing after the critical incident, such as death by suicide. Policy should be developed to support staff and minimize vicarious trauma.
21. Organizations allocate resources to ensure that all nurses have opportunities for clinical supervision and coaching on an ongoing basis.
22. Organizations implement policies regarding the systematic documentation of suicide risk assessment.
23. Organizations promote the service available within the organization and community may support the care of adults at risk for suicidal ideation and behavior.
24. Organizations support nurses' opportunities for professional development and mental health nursing.
25. Organizations support research initiatives related to suicide and other mental health issues.
26. Organizations develop a plan for the implementation of best practice guidelines to include an assessment of organizational readiness and barriers to education; involve all members who will contribute to the implementation process; ongoing opportunities for discussion and education to reinforce the importance of best practices; dedication of a qualified individual to provide the facilitation required for the education and implementation process; opportunities for reflection on personal and organizational experience implementing guidelines; strategies for sustainability; and allocation of adequate resources for implementation and sustainability, including organizational and administrative support.

RISK FOR AGGRESSION

The World Health Organization (WHO), the U.S. Department of Labor Occupational Safety and Health Administration (OSHA), National Institute for Occupational Safety and Health (NIOSH), the American Nurses Association (ANA), the American Association of Occupational Health Nurses (AAOHN), and the U.S. Department of Justice (DOJ) all consider workplace violence an issue of concern. Although more research exists pertaining to acts of aggression in psychiatric settings, in reality aggression can occur in any setting. The DOJ and the Bureau of Labor Statistics (BLS) are the entities that gather statistical data related to this problem. Data from these two sources indicate that health care workers are at increased risk to be victims of workplace violence. BLS reports that there were 69 homicides in health services from 1996 to 2000, and in 2000, 48% of all nonfatal injuries of occupational assault occurred in health care and social services.[17] A study (N = 3465) that looked at incidence of violence against nurses working in U.S. EDs found 25% of participants reported experiencing physical silence more than 20 times in the past 3 years, and almost 20% reported experiencing verbal abuse more than 200 times in the same time period.[18] Workplace violence is an act in which a person is abused, threatened, intimidated, or assaulted in the course of his or her employment. The acts of workplace violence can range from an angry verbal attack to physical assault.[9]

PREVENTION IS KEY

One of the most important things about aggression is to "see it coming." There may be some instances when a person will go from "zero to a hundred" in a few seconds but that is probably rare. The more likely scenario is that there will be multiple opportunities to observe behaviors that signal distress, and early recognition provides opportunity for early intervention. It was established at the beginning of this article that high-dependency environments are very stressful and therefore the people in them are stressed as well.

The Relationship Between Aggression, Anger, and Anxiety

Aggression and anger are closely related. What is more difficult to conceptualize is the relationship between anger and anxiety. Understanding this relationship provides a better opportunity for early intervention and therefore an opportunity to de-escalate potential aggressive incidents. The result of feeling anxious is frustration and helplessness. These feelings in turn cause some individuals to feel powerless to control their own autonomy. Anger is a more powerful feeling than anxiety, particularly in situations in which the person perceives little control. As anxiety brings feelings of helplessness, anger makes people feel better because they feel they have regained some control. In other words, for some people, the intolerable feeling of anxiety is replaced with the more powerful feeling of anger. Although this can be effective as a temporary coping mechanism, it is not very helpful when it is the only coping mechanism that is at a person's disposal.[19]

The open expression of anger is often discouraged and causes others to feel uncomfortable. Anger is a natural emotion and the rational expression of angry feelings can be appropriate for some situations. For example, someone misplacing diagnostic tests of a patient, resulting in the need to repeat the test is probably grounds for some legitimate anger. In these types of situations the person's anger needs to be validated. Nurses are sometimes the recipients of anxious/angry feelings and it is can be difficult for them not to personalize their response to these expressions of emotion with anger of their own. This is particularly true when the focus of the anger is unwarranted. Of course, responding with anger will only serve to escalate the angry feelings.[19] Understanding that increasing anxiety can trigger angry responses provides an opportunity to intervene to decrease anxiety, which is safer and more productive than intervening in an aggressive incident.

If a nurse is confronted with an angry patient or family member, it is imperative to address their concerns. It is important to pick up the early signs of anger because angry feelings tend to increase if the cause for the anger is not addressed. Early intervention to reduce anger and accompanying anxiety increases the probability of a positive outcome. However, if a patient's expression of anger is not rationale or escalating rapidly, the nurse will need to set clear limits and escalate his or her interventions.[19]

Box 4			
Gradation of anger behaviors			
Mild	**Moderate**	**Severe**	**Rage**
• Feeling of tension	• Increasing rumination	• Signs of acting out behavior	• Rage is an out-of-control situation and appropriate interventions to protect the safety of the patient and staff must be implemented immediately
• Feeling irritable	• Angry behavior more obvious	• Cursing	
• Argumentative	• Motor agitation	• Distinct danger of becoming out of control	
• Difficult to please	• Voice pitch increases		
• Scowling facial expression	• Potential for acting out behavior		
• Sarcasm			

Data from Rittenmeyer L. Psychosocial nursing. In Osborn KS, Wraa CE, Watson AB. Medical Surgical Nursing: Preparation for Practice. Boston: Pearson; 2009.

ASSESSMENT AND INTERVENTION

Anger can be conceptualized on a continuum ranging from mild, to moderate, to severe, to rage. **Box 4** illustrates a gradation of anger behaviors.

As indicated earlier, when anxiety or anger is escalating, immediate intervention is required. **Box 5** illustrates interventions.

SYSTEM RESPONSIBILITIES IN REDUCING WORKPLACE VIOLENCE

The Occupational Safety and Health Act (OSHA) of 1970 mandates that employers have a general duty to provide their employees with a hazard-free workplace. Joint Commission Performance Standard EP4 states that hospitals/organizations must have a code of conduct that defines acceptable and disruptive and inappropriate behavior, and performance standard EP 5 states that leaders need to create and implement a process for managing disruptive and inappropriate behavior. In 2004, OSHA published the Guidelines for Preventing Workplace Violence for Healthcare and Social Service Workers. The goal of this guideline is to eliminate or reduce worker exposure to conditions that lead to death or injury from violence by implementing effective security devices and administrative work practices, among other control measures.[20] The following are the major recommendations of the OSHA guideline:

1. Management commitment and employee involvement

Management commitment and employee involvement are complementary and essential elements of an effective safety and health program.

To ensure an effective program, management and frontline employees must work together, perhaps through a team or committee approach.[20]

Box 5		
Nursing interventions for a continuum of anger behaviors		
Prevention	Mild–Moderate	Severe to Rage
• Listen when patients talk to you.	• Help the patient verbalize angry feelings.	• Prevent physical harm to the patient or staff.
• Do not dismiss people's concerns.	• Validate the patient's anger.	• Help the patient identify the source of anger.
• Treat each patient as an individual.	• Avoid defensive responses.	• Support the patient in attempts to control anger.
• Talk to patients, not at them.	• Use therapeutic communication skills.	• Implement a violence code if necessary.
• Respect patients' privacy.	• Assist the patient to identify the source of anger.	
• Don't make rules that treat adults as children.	• Allow the patient an outlet for angry feelings.	
• Recognize when patients are feeling anxious and intervene to reduce the anxiety.	• Engage in mutual problem solving.	
	• Allow the patient more control over health care decisions.	
	• Limit exposure to frustrating situations.	
	• Teach the patient relaxation techniques such as deep breathing.	
	• Continually monitor for possible escalation to a higher level.	

2. Worksite analysis

A worksite analysis involves a step-by-step, commonsense look at the workplace to find existing or potential hazards for workplace violence. This entails reviewing specific procedures or operations that contribute to hazards and specific areas where hazards may develop. A threat assessment team, patient assault team, similar task force, or coordinator may assess the vulnerability to workplace violence and determine the appropriate preventive actions to be taken. This group may also be responsible for implementing the workplace violence prevention program. The team should include representatives from senior management, operations, employee assistance, security, occupational safety and health, legal and human resources staff.[20]

3. Focus of a worksite analysis

The recommended program for worksite analysis includes, but is not limited to:
■ Analyzing and tracking records
■ Screening surveys
■ Analyzing workplace security.[20]

4. Hazard prevention and control

After hazards are identified through the systematic worksite analysis, the next step is to design measures through engineering or administrative and work practices to prevent or control these hazards. If violence does occur, post-incident response can be an important tool in preventing future incidents.[20]

5. Safety and health training

Training and education ensure that all staff are aware of potential security hazards and how to protect themselves and their coworkers through established policies and procedures.[20]

6. Elements of a program evaluation

As part of their overall program, employers should evaluate their safety and security measures. Top management should review the program regularly, and with each incident, to evaluate its success. Responsible parties (including managers, supervisors, and employees) should reevaluate policies and procedures on a regular basis to identify deficiencies and take corrective action. More in-depth guidance may be found at www.OSHA.gov/.

SUMMARY

High-dependency environments are complex both from the standpoint of diversity of patient types and the nature of their functioning. Nurses manage this complexity at many different levels. Being attuned not only to the physical status of the patient but also the emotional/psychological status is paramount in maintaining a safe environment. Staff training and education is paramount in reducing risk. Institutions have a responsibility to provide resources to develop violence prevention programs.[18]

REFERENCES

1. Corr M. Reducing occupational stress in intensive care. Nurs Crit Care 2000;5(2): 76–81.
2. Jozuit D. Suffering of critical care nurses with end-of-life decisions. MEDSURG Nurs 2000;9(3):145–53.
3. Mealer M, Shelton A, Berg B, et al. Increased prevalence off post traumatic stress disorder symptoms in critical care nurses. Am J Respir Crit Care Med 2007;175(7): 693–7.
4. Cuthbertson B, Hull A, Strachan M, et al. Post-traumatic stress disorder after critical illness requiring general intensive care. Intensive Care Med 2003;30(3):450–5.
5. The Joint Commission. A follow-up report on preventing suicide: focus on medical surgical/nursing and the emergency department. Sentinel event alert 2010; Issue 46. Available at: http://www.jointcommission.org/SentinelEvents/. Accessed November 11, 2011.
6. Mills D, Watts B, Vince B, et al. A checklist to identify inpatient suicide hazards in veterans affairs hospitals. Jt Comm J Qual Patient Saf 2010;36(2):87–93.
7. Bostwick J, Rackley S. Completed suicide in medical/surgical patients: who is at risk? Curr Psychiatry Rep 2007;9:242–6.
8. Tischler C, Reiss N. Inpatient suicide: preventing a common sentinel event. Gen Hosp Psychatiry 2009;31:103–9.
9. Agency for Healthcare Research and Quality. Never events. Available at: www.ahrq.gov. Accessed November 11, 2011.
10. The Joint Commission. Sentinel events statistics. Available at: http://www.jointcommission.org/SentinelEvents/. Accessed November 11, 2011.

11. The Joint Commission. Inpatient suicides: recommendations for prevention. Sentinel event alert 1998; Issue 7. Available at: http://www.jointcommission.org/Sentinel Events/. Accessed November 11, 2011.
12. Viilo K, Timononen M, Hakko H, et al. Lifetime prevalence of physical diseases and mental disorders in young suicide victims. Psychosom Med 2005;67:241–5.
13. Cheng A, Chen T, Chen C, et al. Psychosocial and psychiatric risk factors for suicide: case-control autopsy study. Br J Psychiatry 2000;177:360–5.
14. Cheng I, Hu F, Tseng M. Inpatient suicide in a general hospital. Gen Hosp Psychiatry 2009:31;110–5.
15. U.S. Department of Health and Human Services, Public Health Service. National strategy for suicide prevention: goals and objectives for action. Rockville (MD): U.S. Department of Health and Human Services, Public Health Service; 2011.
16. Registered Nurses' Association of Ontario (RNAO). Assessment and care of adults at risk for suicidal ideation and behavior. Toronto (ON): National Guideline Clearinghouse. Available at: www.guideline.gov. Accessed November 11, 2011.
17. U.S. Department of Labor, Bureau of Labor Statistics. Survey of occupational injuries and illnesses 2000, 2001. Available at: www.bls.gov/. Accessed January 15, 2011.
18. Gacki-Smith J, Juarez A, Boyett L. Violence against nurses working in US emergency department. J Nurs Admin 2009;39(7/8):340–9.
19. Rittenmeyer L. Psychosocial Nursing. In: Osborn K, Wraa C, Watson A, editors. Medical Surgical Nursing: Preparation for Practice. (NJ): Pearson; 2009. p. 251–71.
20. U.S. Department of Labor and Occupational Safety and Health Administration. Guidelines for preventing workplace violence for healthcare and social service workers (no. OSHA 3148-1R) 2004. Available at: www.OSHA.gov/. Accessed November 11, 2011.

Incorporating the Treatment of Medical and Psychiatric Disorders in the Critical Care Area

Kathleen L. Patusky, MA, PhD, RN, CNS[a],*, Barbara Caldwell, PhD, APN[a],
David Unkle, MSN, RN, APN, FCCM[a,b], Bruce Ruck, PharmD, DABAT[a,c]

KEYWORDS

- Medical psychiatric comorbidity • Medical psychiatric integration
- Critical care • Intensive care • Comorbidity

Placing the treatment of psychiatric issues on the back burner while acute and critical medical disorders are addressed is not practicable. Too often the behavioral symptoms can interfere with care. The altered demographic and diagnostic categories of critical care patients dictate the need for an increased knowledge base among critical care staff in multiple areas of synthesis between medical and psychiatric care. For most individuals, hospitalization and critical care admission are unusual, generally frightening, experiences. However, critical care nurses must also be prepared to address psychopathologies that present or emerge from a variety of sources.

ATOPIC DISEASE

Although the neuroendocrine response to stress is well documented, the interaction between this response and behavior, immunologic dysfunction, overall state of health, and atopic disease has gained attention only recently. The fields of psychoneuroallergology (PNA) and psychoneurimmunology (PNI) have established links between the physiologic response to stress and its resultant impact on neurobehavioral and immunologic response. Either through stimulation of the hypothalamic–pituitary–adrenal axis (HPAA) or the sympathetic and parasympathetic nervous systems, the end result is activation of immunomodulation pathways that result in

The authors have nothing to disclose.

[a] Graduate Programs, School of Nursing, University of Medicine & Dentistry of New Jersey, 65 Bergen Street, Newark, NJ 07101, USA

[b] Acute/Critical Care Nurse Practitioner Program, School of Nursing, University of Medicine & Dentistry of New Jersey, 40 East Laurel Road, Stratford, NJ 08084, USA

[c] New Jersey Poison Information and Education System, New Jersey Medical School, University of Medicine & Dentistry of New Jersey, 65 Bergen Street, Newark, NJ 07101, USA

* Corresponding author.

E-mail address: patuskkl@umdnj.edu

Crit Care Nurs Clin N Am 24 (2012) 53–80
doi:10.1016/j.ccell.2012.01.001
0899-5885/12/$ – see front matter © 2012 Elsevier Inc. All rights reserved.

adrenocorticotrophic hormone (ACTH) and corticotrophic-releasing hormones. Other hormones released include acetylcholine, epinephrine, norepinephrine, vasopressin, bradykinin, somatostatin, substance P, vasoactive intestinal peptide (VIP) and calcitonin G-related peptide (CGRP), prostaglandins, as well as a number of the interleukins.

Histamine, often the "forgotten neurotransmitter" among the four aminergic systems (histaminergic, dopaminergic, serotonergic, and noradrenergic), is known to activate the sympathetic nervous system and warrants strong consideration in the evaluation of behavior and neuroimmune disorders in both the in-patient and out-patient settings. The relationship between histamine, atopic disease, and behavior has garnered varying degrees of attention with surprising results. Histamine-mediated atopic disease has been linked to migraines and seizure disorders. The coexistence of atopic disease among patients with depression compared to patients with nondepressive psychiatric disorders or control subjects has been reported.[1] An increased incidence of known risk factors for suicide in patients with atopic disease compared to the general population has been noted; the incidence of depression was higher in the suicidal population.[2] Patients with atopic dermatitis were shown to have increased sensory hypersensitivity manifested as labile emotions, hostility, anxiety, and neuroticism.[3,4] Heleniak and O'Desky[5] explored the connection between histamine and prostaglandin release in the etiology of schizophrenia and suggested that abnormal levels of histamine, not dopamine, accounted for the neurobiological changes in patients with schizophrenia. In a systematic review of 43 studies, a robust etiologic and prognostic effect on atopic disease was found.[6] A statistically significant association between seasonal allergic rhinitis and suicidal ideation without attempts has been demonstrated.[7] The fields of PNA and PNI hold promise for additional findings in the future.

ASTHMATIC DISEASE

Among the initial reports establishing the connection between psychological factors and asthmatic disease was MacKenzie's (1886)[8] in his seminal work, "The Production of Rose Asthma by an Artificial Rose." Since that time, asthma has been considered a psychosomatic illness.

Researchers identified a strong relationship between anxiety, depression, and low Asthma Control Test (ACT) scores reflective of poorly controlled asthma.[9] This may be due in part to low ACT scores and poorly controlled asthma serving as an etiology for increased anxiety and depression; or psychological symptoms may heighten awareness of symptoms and be perceived to be worse than actual physiologic function.[10] In patients with severe asthma, morbidity and asthma-related health care costs were more closely related to psychological dysfunction rather than pulmonary function.[11] The relationship between mental illness and asthmatic disease extends beyond the traditional realm. Cookson and colleagues[12] looked at maternal anxiety during pregnancy and its impact on later development of asthma in their children. A longitudinal study of 5810 children revealed that maternal anxiety during pregnancy resulted in the development of asthma in children at 7½ years of age.

PATIENTS WITH PSYCHOPATHOLOGY

Patients may be admitted to the critical care area with a psychopathology, **or** a psychopathology may emerge during the course of treatment (**Table 1**). The aging population, particularly at risk, brings with it dementias, delirium, and late-onset psychiatric disorders that can affect the ability to participate in care effectively or at

Table 1 Patients with potential psychopathology	
Older adults	Dementias, delirium, preexisting psychopathology, late-onset psychiatric disorders
Patients with preexisting history	Mood disorders (depression, bipolar disorder), psychoses (schizophrenia), anxiety disorders (panic disorder, posttraumatic stress disorder, obsessive–compulsive disorder, agoraphobia), substance use disorders
Medication-induced disorders	Serotonin syndrome, neuroleptic malignant syndrome, metabolic syndrome, hypothyroidism, cardiac conduction abnormalities, steroid induced psychosis. Substance-induced delirium, substance-induced dementia, substance-induced amnestic disorder, substance-induced psychotic disorder, substance-induced mood disorder, substance-induced anxiety disorder, substance-induced sexual dysfunction, substance-induced sleep disorder, medication-induced movement disorders[13]
Psychomimetic disorders	NMDA receptor antagonists such as phencyclidine, ketamine, and MK-801 produce schizophrenia-like psychosis; other side effects associated with ketamine are increased blood pressure, diplopia, confusion, dizziness, nystagmus, cardiac arrhythmias, and nausea and vomiting. Alpha-2 adrenergic agonists can cause sedation and sympathetic inhibition.[67]
TRIAD: Medical/psychiatric/ neurologic disorder combination	Erectile dysfunction, depression, and ischemic heart disease[68]; tremor, seizures, and psychosis presenting in chronic lyme borrelliosis; in second stage of the disease Bannwarth's syndrome, cranial neuritis, encephalitis, and transverse myelitis[69]; Charles Bonnet syndrome (CBS) (complex visual hallucinations, ocular pathology causing visual deterioration and preserved cognitive status)–cognitive impairment, stroke, and early Alzheimer's disease may be associated with CBS[70]; auditory, visual, and corticospinal track degeneration (rapidly progressive senorineural hearing loss, blindness, dysarthria, dysphagia, and tetraparesis) in human immunodeficiency virus (HIV) infection[71]

all. The dementias are not limited to Alzheimer's disease (AD). Delirium is particularly essential to diagnose because it is reversible (see article on delirium by Holly and colleagues elsewhere in this issue). Other psychiatric disorders, most commonly emerging at specific life stages, can also appear for the first time at an older age.

The mentally ill population, once consigned to state hospitals, more often is aging In the community and is navigating the health care system at large. Individuals have the potential of needing critical care while in or at risk of major psychiatric episodes. Behavioral and mental status indicators of such an episode may be evident and potentially misinterpreted on admission. Indicators may also emerge after admission, especially if psychiatric medications have not been continued upon admission. Notice of behavioral or mental status changes a few days after admission should automatically trigger a review of potential past psychiatric history and medications. Medication-induced psychopathology or psychomimetic disorders may emerge at any point in hospitalization.

Perhaps the most difficult situation is one the authors have labeled the TRIAD—a medical disorder (eg, congestive heart failure) combined with a psychiatric disorder (eg, bipolar disorder) combined with a neurologic disorder (eg, dementia), discussed later. Managing any of these patients can greatly challenge the critical care system.

DSM-IV-TR

Psychiatric clinicians do not follow the ICD-9 or ICD-10 in the diagnosis of psychiatric disorders. Rather, the *Diagnostic and Statistical Manual of Psychiatric Disorders*, 4th edition, text revision (DSM-IV-TR)[13] provides algorithms that specify the diagnostic criteria for each identified disorder and its subtypes, along with numerical identifiers that differ from those assigned in the ICD. The algorithms are meant to be used as guidelines, and their limitations are recognized. A new edition, the DSM-V, is scheduled for release in 2013, and substantial changes in our current guidelines for disorders, based on research and expert testimony, will be adopted.

A DSM-IV-TR–based diagnosis is noted along five axes. Axis I identifies major psychiatric disorders. Axis II notes personality disorders or mental retardation. Axis III lists general medical conditions. Axis IV identifies psychosocial and environmental problems, such as poverty or divorce. Axis V is the Global Assessment of Functioning (GAF), graded from 0 to 100. The numbers assigned by the clinician are meant to depict current functioning based on the degree to which symptoms interfere with life activities. The following are examples of a DSM diagnosis:

Axis I - 296.23 Major Depressive Disorder, Single Episode, Severe without Psychotic Features

Axis II – 301.9 Personality Disorder NOS (not otherwise specified)

Axis III – Newly diagnosed breast cancer; hypothyroidism

Axis IV – Insufficient health insurance, social isolation

Axis V – GAF 50 (meaning serious impairment in functioning with few friends)

The following sections address normal responses to the critical care area and each of the relevant adult areas of the DSM-IV-TR, providing the diagnostic criteria, differential diagnoses, primary treatments, and other limited information. In some instances, brief case studies describe presentations of the psychiatric diagnosis with medical disorders.

NORMAL RESPONSES TO THE CRITICAL CARE AREA

Consider the impact experienced by individuals without a medical background who are admitted to critical care areas under emergency conditions. Fear, anxiety, and confusion can be expected, with greater awareness of the environment only once the emergent phase has passed. Multiple studies have identified anxiety, depression, and posttraumatic stress as potential problems,[14,15] with some patients experiencing frightening memories of critical care.[16,17] Patients on mechanical ventilation have demonstrated patterns of highly individualized anxiety, varying over time and not dependent upon sedative use.[18] A recent study has suggested that depressive symptoms may trigger cardiac complications (eg, ischemia, cardiac arrest), necessitating early identification and treatment of emotional symptoms.[19] Comparisons of anxiety, depression, and posttraumatic stress after intensive care discharge showed that these psychological symptoms had not decreased significantly over time, even at 9 months later.[20,21] Further, at hospital discharge patients' perceptions of their intensive care experience was significantly associated with their symptom scores.[20]

The impact of the critical care experience extends beyond the point of hospital discharge.

DELIRIUM, DEMENTIA, AND AMNESTIC AND OTHER COGNITIVE DISORDERS

As stated, the dementias are not limited to Alzheimer's disease. They include vascular (multi-infarct) dementia; dementia related to Parkinson's disease; and dementia associated with Lewy body disease, Pick's disease, and other frontal lobe dementias. Other medical conditions that can present with dementia are brain tumors, subdural hematoma, head trauma, and endocrine conditions.[22] **Table 2** describes the onset, DSM criteria, differential diagnosis, and treatment for the main disorders in this category.

Intensive care unit (ICU) delirium has been reported—most commonly hypoactive and mixed types. Sleep disruption due to ambient noise and lighting has been suggested as a possible risk factor in ICU delirium.[23-25] Although delirium might also be due to preexisting cognitive impairment or other medical precipitants, in one case study no organic etiology was found. The authors described a woman with a death anxiety who developed delirium, and suggested that ICU delirium might be considered psychosomatic—either a stress response after surgery or a defense against death anxiety. No other cause was ever found.[26]

SCHIZOPHRENIA AND OTHER PSYCHOTIC DISORDERS

Not all psychotic states indicate schizophrenia. Many street drugs as well as prescribed medications can result in psychosis. Use of amphetamines or phencyclidine (PCP) can cause schizophrenia-type symptoms or trigger relapse in someone who does have schizophrenia. A single dose of an N-methyl-D-aspartate (NMDA) receptor antagonist, such as ketamine, can also result in schizophrenia-like symptoms.[27] Although symptoms may be similar, schizophrenia is a chronic disorder with periodic remissions. Removal of a causal agent, time, and appropriate medication may be sufficient to address symptoms of a brief psychotic reaction. However, follow-up would be needed to determine if the patient has returned to usual functioning, or if a stage of schizophrenia has been reached. Schizophrenia has been described in acute, stabilization, and stable stages. Remission of symptoms changes to a focus on minimizing risk of relapse because succeeding episodes can result in increasing residual symptoms.[28] **Table 3** addresses additional information on the psychoses.

An episode of substance-induced psychosis serves as a differentiation from schizophrenia. In a Southern California hospital, two men in their early 20s were admitted via the emergency room to the psychiatric unit. They were in an advanced state of confusion and disorganization, with active visual hallucinations, hyperthermia, and tachycardia. For their own safety, they were placed in totally empty unlocked seclusion rooms with close observation. The degree of their hallucinations was apparent, as one man acted as if he were typing on a nonexistent typewriter, and the other urinated in a nonexistent commode. They might have been considered schizophrenic: male, early adulthood, disorganized, hallucinating. But other elements did not fit: coming in together with the same symptoms, no apparent prodromal profile, visual rather than auditory hallucinations. Add to these elements the fact that the men were found in a desert area where jimson weed ("loco weed" or *datura stramonium*) was known to grow, and the diagnosis became anticholinergic psychosis. Two doses of physotigmine given to each man reversed the symptoms completely, with typical amnesia for the period of delirium.

Table 2
Delirium, dementia, and amnestic and other cognitive disorders

Diagnosis	Onset	DSM Criteria	Differential Diagnosis	Treatments
Delirium—due to medical condition	Normally develops over hours but can develop abruptly	• Disturbance in consciousness with inability to maintain or change focus • Changes in cognition such as memory problems, disorientation, articulation problems or perceptual changes • History, physical examination, or laboratory test changes present	Dementia, substance intoxication or withdrawal, brief psychotic disorder, schizophrenia, mood disorder with psychotic features, acute stress reaction[13] Infection, cardiovascular disease, cerebrovascular disease, metabolic diseases, head trauma, epilepsy, brain tumor, poisoning, extensive life stress	• Main goal is to establish cause of the delirium. • Treatment is empirical and few guidelines are noted. • Support systems • Fluid and electrolyte balance • Prevent urinary obstruction. • Manage gastrointestinal (GI) system. • Discontinue all unnecessary medication. • Adequate lighting and familiar objects • Addition of scheduled quetiapine to as-needed haloperidol results in faster resolution of delirium, decreased time in delirium, and less agitation.[73] • Foster sleep and if necessary, zopiclone 3.75–7.5 mg hs. • Opiates and benzodiazepines are associated with increased risk of developing delirium in the elderly.[74] • Excited delirium syndrome: Clinical features include acute drug intoxication, usually attributed to cocaine.

				• Aggressive and erratic behaviors involving law enforcement and use of TASERS • Better education of EMS and law enforcement[75] • Delirium prevention[76]

Amnestic disorders	Variable depending on the underlying pathology	• Impaired ability to learn new information, recall previously acquired information or past events
		• Memory must cause serious impairment to social and occupational functioning
		• Serious reduction in previous level of functioning.
			Delirium, dementia, dissociative disorders, substance intoxication or withdrawal, malingering, and factitious disorder
			Transient ischemic attack (TIA), brain injuries, epileptic seizures, medications, stimulants, depression, hypothyroidism, hyper- and hypocalcaemia, vitamin B deficiency, infections, hypoglycemia and psychosis[72]
				• Treat underlying pathology.
				• Drug therapy based on behavioral profile and in low doses and short periods in the elderly can include benzodiazepines, antipsychotic drugs, antidepressant drugs, anticholinesterases, and memantine and drugs for insomnia[77]
				• Factors that contribute to increasing memory problems:
				  ○ Being alone for a prolonged time
				  ○ Increased stimuli
				  ○ Darkness (suitable lighting also at nighttime
				  ○ All infections (urinary infection is the most common)
				  ○ Hot weather (heat, fluid loss)
				  ○ Extensive medication.
				  ○ Behavioral management

(continued on next page)

Table 2 *(continued)*				
Diagnosis	Onset	DSM Criteria	Differential Diagnosis	Treatments
Dementia of the Alzheimer's type	Progressive, static, or remitting course based on etiology	• Cognitive deficits • Memory impairment • Aphasia • Apraxia • Agnosia • Treat pain, dehydration, and constipation. • Distubance in executive functioning • Significant impairment in social or occupational functioning	Delirium; amnestic disorder; vascular dementia; substance intoxication; mental retardation; schizophrenia; major depression; malingering or factitious disorder; cardiovascular disease; Parkinson disease; Huntington's disease; subdural hematoma; brain tumor; hypothyroidism; vitamin B_{12}, folic acid, or niacin deficiency; human immunodeficiency virus (HIV); hypercalcemia; neurosyphilis	• Review medications to avoid polypharmacy and discontinue unnecessary medications. • Assess cognitive function every 8 hours (MMSE, Mini-Cog) and make appropriate referrals to a multidisciplinary team trained in delirium prevention.[78] • Avoid changing surroundings or staff. • Reorientation with use of clocks, calendars, lighting, and family visits • Treat pain, dehydration, and constipation. • Optimize oxygen saturation.

- Evaluate for infections and avoid unnecessary catheterization.
- Encourage early mobility and assess reversible causes of hearing and visual impairment.
- Avoid sleep disturbance.[73]
- Opiates and benzodiazepines are associated with an increased risk of developing delirium in elderly hospitalized patients:
  - Balance relief of pain against the risk of delirium.[74]
  - Control restlessness with risperidone 0.25–0.5 mg
  - Can be at increased risk of death and cardiovascular events.[65]
  - Low-dose haloperidol in severe agitation but caution with dementia patients
  - Can precipitate extrapyramidal adverse reactions.

(continued on next page)

Table 2
(continued)

Diagnosis	Onset	DSM Criteria	Differential Diagnosis	Treatments
				• Use of cholinesterase inhibitors (ChEIs; tacrine, donepezil, rivastigmine, and galantamine) as the standard of care in Alzheimer's disease; and effective with psychosis and agitation[79]
Vascular dementia	Abrupt with fluctuating course with rapid changes in patient level of functioning	• Same as above but has focal neurologic symptoms: exaggerated deep tendon reflex, extensor plantar reflex, pseudobulbar palsy, gait and extremity weakness or laboratory results that indicate cortical infarcts		• See above. • Support for the use of donepezil in improving cognition function, clinical global impression, and activities of daily living in patients with probable or possible mild to moderate vascular cognitive[80]

MOOD DISORDERS

Mood disorders are especially complex, as uncontrolled highs and lows of mood may be masked; may be singular or recurrent; and may change over months, years, or within the same day. Mood disorders must meet the standards of the DSM-IV guidelines. Such disorders do not include normal sadness or bereavement over a loss or disappointment, although prolonged mood disturbance should be evaluated; they do not include euphoria over hearing positive medical news. However, depression in particular is more prevalent in persons with chronic medical conditions, everything from cardiac disease to diabetes mellitus and beyond.[29] In fact, an extensive scientific review of the literature assessed the effect of mood disorders on selected medical comorbidities and suggested there might be biological mechanisms accounting for the links found. The authors recommended further studies as well as clinical policy changes to screen all medical patients for depression and to be prepared to treat depression early.[30] See **Table 4** for additional details on mood disorders.

Depression has been noted to play a major role after both stroke and myocardial infarction (MI),[31-33] with some differences in presentation. Stroke patients showed more loss of interest, psychomotor retardation, and gastrointestinal discomfort,[31] no doubt affecting ability to participate in care. Depression seemed to have a greater influence on stroke patients, as their reported Quality of Life (QOL) was worse in patients after stroke than the reported QOL of post-MI patients.[34] However, the combination of depression and low social support has been shown to be associated with greater risk affecting recovery after an MI.[35] According to one researcher, the existence of depression before an MI was a significant independent predictor of all complications that occurred in intensive care except ischemia on multiple regression analysis.[36] Post-MI depression increased cardiac mortality.[37] Given the aforementioned findings, the need to evaluate patients for depression becomes clear.

ANXIETY DISORDERS

The category of anxiety disorders comprises a number of seemingly disparate diagnoses, including agoraphobia, panic disorder, specific phobias, social phobia, obsessive–compulsive disorder, posttraumatic stress disorder (PTSD), acute stress disorder, generalized anxiety disorder, and anxiety disorder due to a medical disorder or substance use.[13] Apart from PTSD, studies of anxiety in critical care areas have focused mostly on state anxiety rather than specific diagnoses. See **Table 5** for details about some anxiety disorders.

As noted earlier, anxiety and posttraumatic stress have been identified in response to the critical care experience,[14,15,20,21] and patients on ventilators are at particular risk for anxiety.[18] Higher anxiety and depression can be seen among elderly cardiac patients, but should not be viewed as a function of aging.[38] Nurses' caring behavior is important to relieve fear and worry.[39] In two studies with cardiovascular surgery patients, 20 minutes of massage between postoperative days 2 and 5 decreased pain, anxiety, and tension.[40,41] However, the nurse should be aware that even if anxiety levels are decreased during the intensive care stay, there is an increased risk of transfer anxiety with women, with people having lower social support, and with patients who have had a longer ICU stay.[42]

Otherwise healthy Veterans Administration patients with depression, anxiety disorder nos, panic disorder, or PTSD were found to be at greater risk for MI.[32] Anxiety and anxiety comorbid with depression are risk indicators for coronary artery disease.[43] After an acute MI, anxiety is common, increasing complications and length of stay. Beta blockers have been tried and were found to be ineffective in decreasing the

Table 3
Schizophrenia and other psychotic disorders

Diagnosis	Onset	DSM Criteria	Differential Diagnosis	Treatments
Schizophrenia— Can be subtypes: • Paranoid • Disorganized • Catatonic • Undifferentiated • Residual	First episode is in 20s with either a rapid or slow course with prodromal symptoms such as social isolation, loss of interest in persons and surroundings, poor hygiene, unusual behaviors.	Within 1 month, the following symptoms develop: • Delusions • Hallucinations • Disorganized speech, thinking, and behavior • Flat or inappropriate affect Lack of interest	Psychotic disorder due to medical condition; substance-induced psychosis; mood disorder with psychotic features; bipolar disorder; delusional disorder; pervasive developmental disorder; schizotypal, schizoid, borderline, or paranoid personality disorder	New onset: • Assessment of etiology • Assess for suicidality and potential for violent behavior. • Implement safety plan to protect patient from harming self or others. • Antipsychotic medication based on potential side effect profiles • Adjunctive drug therapy with mood stabilizers, antidepressants, or benzodiazepines with mood symptoms • Use of soothing music and same staff members • Talk to patient and understand fears. • Discuss current activities in calm manner based on patient's capacity to understand and cope. • Provide psychoeducation with family. • Initiate if possible and refer for CBT. • If patient is being discharged directly home, ensure family members have emergency crisis phone numbers and psychiatric follow-up[81]

Delusional disorder subtypes • Erotomanic • Grandiose • Jealous • Persecutory • Somatic	Variable with remission and progression	• Nonbizarre delusions based on real-life events • No changes in behavior or functioning	Psychotic disorder due to medical condition, substance-induced psychosis, schizophrenia, schizophreniform disorder, mood disorder with psychotic features	Children treated in the ICU have increased risk of PTSD and delusional memories.[82]
Brief psychotic disorder	Onset in 20s and course can be brief in nature	• Delusions • Hallucinations • Disorganized behavior and speech	Psychotic disorder due to medical condition, substance-induced intoxication, schizophreniform disorder, delusional disorder, or mood disorder with psychotic features	See Table 4 under major depressive disorder.

Table 4
Mood disorders

Diagnosis	Onset	DSM Criteria	Differential Diagnosis	Treatments
Major depressive disorder	At least 2 weeks duration and usually develops over days to weeks	• Depressed mood • Loss of interest or pleasure • Significant weight loss or gain • Insomnia or hypersomnia • Psychomotor agitation or retardation • Fatigue or loss of energy • Feelings of worthlessness or guilt that is unwarranted • Recurrent thoughts of death or hurting self	Mood disorder due to medical condition, substance-induced mood disorder, dementia, manic episode with irritable mood, attention-deficit/hyperactivity disorder, adjustment disorder with depressed mood	If admission is related to a suicide attempt, should consider questions such as: • Can you describe what happened? • What did you think would happen? • What thought were you having beforehand that led to the attempt? If a psychotic depression, consider: • Can you describe the voices? What do the voices say? How do you cope with the voices? • Can you describe your thoughts at the time you where thinking about this attempt? • Methods for harm including patient's lethality and expectations • Continued assessment of hopelessness and suicidal ideation[22,83] • Unit safety plan to protect patient and others • CBT[84,85] • Use of SSRI, especially paroxetine in the elderly[86] • Ensure a comprehensive psychiatric plan follow-up in community.

Manic episode	Onset is in adolescents, early 20s or 50s and rapid course with increased symptoms over several days.	Mood elevated or irritable • Inflated self-esteem • Decreased sleep • More talkative than usual • Distractability • Flight of ideas • Increased goal-related activities • Excess in pleasurable activities • Interference with social and occupational functioning	Mood disorder due to medical condition, substance-induced mood disorder, hypomanic episode, attention-deficit/hyperactivity disorder	Continuous assessment of suicidality: • Use of mood stabilizers: carbamazepine, valproic acid, lamotrigine, and atypical antipsychotics (olanzapine and quetiapine)[87] • CBT and psychoeducation[88]
Bipolar I disorder specifiers: • With or without psychotic features • With catatonic features • With melancholic features • With rapid cycling	Onset is 20s.	• Occurrence of one or more manic episodes or mixed episodes • Attempted suicide in 10%–15% of individuals when in a depressed or mixed state	Mood disorder due to medical condition, substance-induced mood disorder, major depressive disorder, dysthymic disorder, psychotic disorder	• Screen for depression, irritability, or impulsivity using a validated instrument. • Assess suicidal ideation, intensity, severity • Has higher incidence of medical comorbidity such as metabolic syndrome and higher cardiovascular risk[89] • Quetiapine and olanzapine-fluoxetine combination showed the greatest symptomatic improvement.[90]
Bipolar II disorder (recurrent major depressive episode with hypomanic episodes)	Occur immediately before or after a major depressive episode; decrease intervals between episodes.	• Presence as noted by history of one or more major depressive episodes (see earlier for major depressive disorder) • One hypomanic episode • No manic episode • Significant distress or impairment in social, occupational function		See above. • Family psychoeducation • CBT (addressing interpersonal problems and regulating emotions)[91]

Table 5
Anxiety disorders

Diagnosis	Onset	DSM Criteria	Differential Diagnosis	Treatments
Panic disorder • With agoraphobia • Without agoraphobia	Onset between adolescence and mid-30s: chronic and intermittent	Unexpected panic attack (period of intense fear or discomfort) with a set of four symptoms as follows: • Heart pounding • Sweating • Shaking • Choking feeling • Chest pain • Nausea or abdominal distress • Dizziness, unsteady gait • Fear of losing control or dying • Numbness • Chills or feeling flushed • Fear or worry of having panic attack	Anxiety disorder due to medical condition, substance-induced anxiety disorder, social phobia, generalized anxiety disorder, PTSD, separation anxiety disorder	• Assess symptoms, functional impairment, and suicidality. • CBT for anxiety[92]
Obsessive–compulsive disorder	Begins in adolescence with acute or chronic onset.	Obsessions: • Recurrent thoughts, impulses, or images that are intrusive and cause anxiety and distress • Attempted suppression of thoughts, images, or impulses • Person understands that they are a product of his or her mind. Compulsions: • Repetitive behaviors person driven to complete based on obsession • Behaviors or mental acts aimed to reduce distress or prevent a dreaded event from happening— no connection and excessive • Causes marked distress and time consuming (>1 hour per day)	Anxiety disorder due to medical condition, substance-induced anxiety disorder, social phobia, generalized anxiety disorder, hypochondriasis, delusional or psychotic disorder, tic disorder, eating disorder, pathologic gambling, obsessive–compulsive personality disorder	• Use validated instrument to confirm diagnosis. • CBT and medication are effective. Can include exposure to anxiety-arousing obsessions while interrupting compulsions. • If prescribing an SSRI, start with half using starting dose and titrate upward depending on response and side effects that occur.[93]

| PTSD | Can occur at any age and start after a traumatic event—can be acute or chronic. | • Exposure, witnessed or experienced a traumatic event
• Intense fear, helplessness or horror (may be agitated or disorganized)
• Recurrent and intrusive thoughts of event
• Recurrent dream of the event
• Sense of reliving the event
• Extreme psychological distress when thinking of the event or something that resembles the event
• Physiological reactivity
• Avoidance of the stimuli concerning the traumatic event
• Numbing
• Inability to recall event
• Feelings of detachment
• Restrict range of affect
• Sense of shortened future
• Increased arousal (sleep problems, irritability, problems concentrating, hypervigilance, increased startle reflex
• Significant impairment in social or occupational function. | Adjustment disorder, acute stress disorder, obsessive–compulsive disorder, schizophrenia, psychotic disorders, mood disorder with psychotic features | Therapeutic working relationship
Use of SSRIs and serotonin–norepinephrine reuptake inhibitors (SNRIs)
Prazosin 3–15 mg
CBT
EMDR[94] |

anxiety.[44] Post-MI anxiety has been found to be linked with a 36% increase in the risk for adverse cardiac outcomes,[45] for recurrent events, and for complications.[36,46] One reason may be that clinical anxiety (having a diagnosed disorder rather than state) was found to influence parasympathetic modulation of the heart rate negatively post-MI.[47] Addressing the anxiety is an important intervention; anxiety during hospitalization and 4 months later has been associated with lower adherence to multiple risk-reducing health behaviors after MI, including such behaviors as following a diet, exercising regularly, decreasing stress, and increasing socialization.[48]

More PTSD symptoms are seen with coronary artery bypass grafting and angioplasty.[49] In such cases, the use of cognitive–behavioral therapy (CBT) may be helpful. Patients' perceived consequences and dysfunctional coping may respond to the CBT techniques that are aimed at changing negative cognitions.[50]

A special word should be mentioned about one more group of patients. High levels of anxiety have been found in 24% to 34% of patients and depression in 14% to 22% of patients, with a history of pacemaker, pacemaker-defibrillator, postcoronary intervention, or atrial fibrillation. Experiencing "shock storm" (greater than or equal to three shocks in a 24-hour period) greatly increased anxiety and resulted in pathologic levels of anxiety. CBT can again be helpful, along with psychoeducation for spouses, and anxiolytic or antidepressant medications may be needed.[51]

SLEEP DISORDERS

Table 6 provides some details about the major sleep disturbance diagnoses. The more we learn about sleep, the more obvious its importance to health. Disturbed sleep in myocardial infarction patients has been associated with anxiety, depression, and fatigue.[52] Sleep disruption in an ICU includes disturbed circadian pattern, prolonged sleep latencies, sleep fragmentation, decreased sleep efficiency, frequent arousals, decreased sleep at night, abnormally increased stages 1 and 2 sleep, reduced or absent deep sleep, and decreased or absent REM sleep.[53,54] Sedation is often used to calm patients or promote sleep, and can contribute to amnesia of ICU occurrences. Still, 57% of patients reported inadequate sleep in one study of sedation. Sedation protocols must be carefully determined and monitored.[55–57] Earplugs may be helpful for unmedicated cardiac patients, but they do not ensure that there is sufficient time for the patient to fall asleep before they will be awakened.[58]

Sleep duration has been found to be an independent risk factor for cardiovascular disease mortality and morbidity in women but not men. The highest risk is at extreme ends of distribution: 6 or 9 hours of sleep.[59,60] In Japanese studies, men who slept less than 6 hours were at risk of cardiovascular events.[61,62] The effect of shortened sleep (≤ 6 hours) was greatest among persons who reported some sleep disturbance.[63] When a patient becomes focused on the need to sleep, that focus sets up a burst of adrenalin and wakefulness continues.[64] Critical care areas are not generally known for permitting restful sleep of any length; yet that is just what patients need.

MEDICATION-INDUCED DISORDERS

Psychotropic medications have as toxic effects some specific disorders, such as serotonin syndrome or neuromuscular malignant syndrome. Medical medications that also affect the serotonin system may cause serotonin syndrome with or without the presence of psychotropic medications. There are so many possible medication issues that they cannot be covered reasonably in this short space. The reader is referred to the article on psychotropic toxicities (Medical and behavioral manifestations following toxic ingestion of psychotropic agents, by Unkle, Ruck, Caldwell, & Patusky). At the same time, it is critical to remember that just about any medication, or any combination of medications, can demonstrate behavioral effects. **Table 1** lists some of them. A better example might be the following case study of an actual occurrence.

AR is a 76-year-old woman admitted to a hospital for difficulty breathing and swallowing secretions secondary to a foreign object (metal plate screw from a surgical procedure) pressing into her esophagus. Initial therapy consisted of high-dose steroids, an attempt to decrease inflammation. On admission she was awake, alert, and oriented. She was living at home with an aide who assisted with physical activities. She was able to perform all mental activates including banking, making appointments, paying rent, and reading.

Forty-eight hours after admission (after several doses of steroids) AR became confused and agitated. Haloperidol was prescribed for the agitation. Over the next 2 days her mental status declined, she was not aware of her surroundings, and she became more agitated and more confused. The family was questioned by the new medical team (which changed every 2 weeks) as to how this patient was really able to function at home. The medical team had not seen the patient on admission, only after she developed the altered mental state. The patient's son (a pharmacist) confirmed that the patient's mental status was "fine" before admission. He suggested that the altered mental status was drug-induced steroid psychosis in conjunction with the haloperidol. After much discussion, haloperidol and steroids were discontinued. The metal screw was removed during a surgical procedure. Within 48 hours of medication discontinuation the patient's mental status was back to baseline with no confusion or agitation. The patient was once again able to perform all previous mental functions and she returned home with an aide for physical assistance only.

TRIAD

The psychiatric discipline has long recognized the combination of a major psychiatric disorder and a substance use disorder as *dual diagnosis*. The authors coin a new term to identify a new medical phenomenon: TRIAD. The TRIAD is the combination of a medical disorder, a psychiatric disorder, and a neurologic disorder in the same individual at a given time. None of these disorders can be specified, and they need not occur singly. Rather, the assessment of a TRIAD must clearly and accurately identify each segment's diagnos(es), with the understanding that each segment can contain multiple diagnoses. Failure to do so opens the door to a myriad of potential problems that could be avoided with an expanded, appropriate knowledge base. The case study in **Box 1** provides an example of how a typical case can spin out of control.

The TRIAD became known to one of the authors during the care of a client receiving home health care visits. A white patient in her 50s was referred by the primary physician because the patient was unwilling to take medications for her newly diagnosed severe hypertension, stating that her body was perfect and she did not need the medication. She had a diagnosis of bipolar disorder and was hypomanic, taking a mood stabilizer each day. Her physician hoped that a psychiatric nurse might be able to convince the patient to be adherent with the new medication. In two home visits over 3 days it became apparent that the client suffered from short-term memory problems and was unable to remember to take medications, initially ordered on a three-times-a-day basis. Further, she would move medications around in her med box, placing her at risk for overdose. Administration of the Folstein Mini-Mental State

Table 6
Sleep disorders

Diagnosis	Onset	DSM Criteria	Differential Diagnosis	Treatments
Primary insomnia	Sudden onset with causative factors	• Difficulty falling and staying asleep • Daytime fatigue—with impairment in social or occupational function	Primary hypersomnia, narcolepsy, breathing related sleep disorder, insomnia related to medical or mental disorder, substance-induced sleep disorder	• Melatonin from 0.1 mg to 10 mg[95] • Use of CBT (50-minute sessions over 6 weeks) with zolipidem[96] (observe for adverse effect such as depression and rebound insomnia) • Eszopiclone and escitalopram in coadministration for anxiety and insomnia[97] (observe for adverse effect such as depression and rebound insomnia)
Primary hypersomnia	Begins between 15 and 30 years with chronic, periodic course	• Excessive sleepiness for at least 1 month • Impairment in social or occupational function	Primary insomnia, narcolepsy, breathing-related sleep disorder, insomnia related to medical or mental disorder, substance -induced sleep disorder, circadian rhythm sleep disorder, bipolar disorder, mood disorder	Treatment options include: • Amphetamine, methamphetamine, dextroamphetamine, and methylphenidate are effective for daytime sleepiness. • Can use short- and long-term forms of stimulants for some patients.[98]
Narcolepsy	Adolescence but history of sleepiness in childhood	• Irresistible attacks of refreshing sleep that occur every day • Cataplexy • Recurrent intrusions of rapid eye movement (REM) into transition between sleep and wakefulness manifested as hypnagogic hallucinations or sleep paralysis	Sleep deprivation, primary hypersomnia, breathing-related sleep disorder, hypersomnia related to another mental disorder, use or withdrawal of substances, sleep disorder due to medical problems	Treatment options include: • Modafinil for daytime sleepiness. • Amphetamine, methamphetamine, dextroamphetamine, and methylphenidate are effective for daytime sleepiness due to narcolepsy. • Scheduled naps[98]

| Breathing-related sleep disorder | Can occur at any age—obstructed airway with gradual progression | • Sleep disruption that is associated with increased sleepiness or insomnia due to sleep apnea | Primary hypersomnia, circadian rhythm sleep disorder, hypersomnia related to major depressive disorder, nocturnal panic attacks, attention-deficit/hyperactivity disorder, withdrawal of substances, sleep disorder due to medical problems | • Use of polysomnography as diagnostic for obstructive sleep apnea
• CPAP with additional support of behavioral therapy, educational intervention, and support groups to increase compliance with treatment [99] |

Box 1
TRIAD case study

A typical older adult admitted to critical care might be diagnosed with congestive heart failure (CHF), renal insufficiency, diabetes, and hypertension. The same individual may have been previously diagnosed with major depression and panic disorder. At the same time, the patient may be constipated, manifested as delirium. In this example, the treatment focus might be centered on breathing difficulties secondary to the CHF, monitoring renal function and hypertension, and maintaining an appropriate blood sugar level. It is also a set of unexpected disasters waiting to happen. Suppose the patient's escitalopram (selective serotonin reuptake inhibitor [SSRI] antidepressant, also used for panic attacks) has not been continued on admission. Constipation is a side effect of the SSRI, but may not be reversed as soon as the medication is stopped.[65] Suppose, also, that the delirium has been misdiagnosed as dementia.

Problem Areas

1. If a serotonergic medication is started for medical purposes while escitalopram is still in the system, serotonin syndrome may result in symptoms of tachycardia or heart rhythm disturbances, hypertension, fever, sweating, shivering, increased confusion, anxiety, tremors, muscle spasms, and rigidity.[66]

2. If a serotonergic medication is not started and the escitalopram is not continued, within a few days the patient may experience a withdrawal from the SSRI. Discontinuation side effects include electrical shocks in the head and/or body (brain shivers), feeling like losing consciousness or actually blacking out, and short-term memory problems.[66] At the same time, the patient's depression symptoms will recur.

3. If the patient has blacked out, or fallen as a result of her agitated delirium, a magnetic resonance imaging scan (MRI) may be ordered. This person with panic disorder may not tolerate a closed MRI, and behavioral symptoms may be assumed to be psychotic. If antipsychotic medications are administered, the constipation is likely to worsen.[65]

4. The constipation has not been treated, so delirium persists. Clinicians insist this is dementia, while the family members are becoming increasingly upset, insisting the patient was not like this at home. (Granted, the family may not have noticed dementia symptoms that were minimized in the familiar setting of home, but highlighted in the confusing ICU setting. On the other hand, the family may be correct.) The disagreement threatens the ability of staff and family members to work together in helping the patient. Placement issues, problems with daily care, and the potential of a chronic delirium are continuing threats, along with untreated constipation, depression, and whatever sequelae are caused by the medical response to unrecognized serotonin syndrome.

What would you do?

Table 1 offers additional possibilities of TRIAD cases.

---

exam demonstrated that the patient likely had early-to-mid stage dementia, masked by her bipolar symptoms.

Treatment of the above patient was not easy, with delusional, irritable, and hypomanic symptoms frequently intruding, and spiking blood pressure a danger. Her strengths included at least average intelligence, an intermittent willingness to listen and learn about her medical situation, a habit of taking her psychotropic medications each morning, and a supportive sister who aided the treatment plan. The physician willingly changed her dosing to twice a day. A visit schedule was constructed that involved gradual decrease from every day to every other day then to less frequent visits, interspersed with phone calls by the nurse to insure morning meds were taken properly. The sister would call or visit each evening to insure the evening med was taken properly. Over time the patient was able to develop the habit of taking medications twice a day with very limited reminders. In this case, building a habit worked; but so many other outcomes could have occurred.

SUMMARY

Critical care areas are fast moving, often chaotic, and therefore confusing, even frightening, to patients attempting to understand what has happened to them. The nurse acts to mitigate these reactions by understanding the range of possibilities that can occur with patients, including potential psychiatric issues, and serving as patient advocate to ensure that appropriate treatment is initiated. Certainly there may be other psychiatric problems not described in the preceding text. The main possibilities are covered in this article. Assessing and acting early are tools the critical care nurse uses to meet patient needs and prevent behavioral problems that can interfere with life-preserving care.

REFERENCES

1. Nasr S, Altman E, Meltzer H. Concordance of allergic and affective disorders. J Affect Disord 1981;291–6.
2. Postolache TT, Komarow H, Tonelli LH. Allergy: a risk factor for suicide? Curr Treat Options Neurol 2008;10:363–76.
3. Engel-Yeger B, Mimouni D, Rozenman, D, et al. Sensory processing patterns of adults with atopic dermatitis. J Eur Acad Dermatol Venerol 2011;25:152–6.
4. Jordan JM, Whittock FA. Emotions and the skin: the conditioning of scratch responses in cases of atopic dermatitis. Br J Dermatol 1972;86:574–85.
5. Heleniak E, O'Desky I. Histamine and prostaglandins in schizophrenia: revisited. Med Hypotheses 1999;52:37–42.
6. Chida Y, Hamer M, Steptoe A. A bidirectional relationship between psychosocial factors and atopic disorders: a systematic review and meta-analysis. Psychosom Med 2008;70:102–16.
7. Messias E, Clarke DR, Goodwin RD. Seasonal allergies and suicidality: results from the National Comorbidity Survey Replication. Acta Psychiatr Scand 2010; 122:139–42.
8. MacKenzie JN. The production of rose asthma by an artificial rose. Am J Med Sci 1886;91:45–57.
9. DiMarco F, Verga M, Santus P, et al. Close correlation between anxiety, depression, and asthma control. Respir Med 2010;104:22–8.
10. Kuehn BM. Asthma linked to psychiatric disorders. JAMA 2008;299:158–60.
11. tenBrinke A, Ouwerkerk ME, Zwinderman AH, et al. Psychopathology in patients with severe asthma is associated with increased health care utilization. Am J Respir Crit Care Med 2001;163:1093–6.
12. Cookson H, Granell R, Johnson C, et al. Mothers' anxiety during pregnancy is associated with asthma in their children. J Allergy Clin Immunol 2009;123:847–53.
13. American Psychiatric Association. Diagnostic and statistical manual of mental disorders, 4th edition, text revision. Washington, DC: American Psychiatric Association; 2000.
14. Cuthbertson BH, Hull A, Strachan M, et al. Post-traumatic stress disorder after critical illness requiring general intensive care. Intensive Care Med 2004;450–5.
15. Rattray J, Johnson M, Wildsmith JAW. Predictors of emotional outcome of intensive care. Anaesthesia 2005;60:1085–92.
16. Jones C, Skirrow P, Griffiths R, et al. Rehabilitation after critical illness: a randomized, controlled trial. Crit Care Med 2003;31:2456–61.

17. Samuelson KAM, Lundberg D, Fridlund B. Stressful memories and psychological distress in adult mechanically ventilated intensive care patients—a 2-month follow-up study. Acta Anaesthesiol Scand 2007;51:671–8.
18. Chlan L, Savik K. Patterns of anxiety in critically ill patients receiving mechanical ventilatory support. Nurs Res 2011;60(3S):S50–7.
19. Grewal K, Stewart DE, Abbey SE, et al. Timing of depressive symptom onset and in-hospital complications among acute coronary syndrome in patients. Psychosomatics 2010;51(4):283–8.
20. Rattray J, Crocker C, Jones M, et al. Patients' perceptions of and emotional outcome after intensive care: results from a multicentre study. Nurs Crit Care 2010;15(2):86–93.
21. Sukantarat K, Greer S, Brett S, et al. Physical and psychological sequelae of critical illness. Br J Health Psychol 2007;12(Pt 1):65–74.
22. American Psychiatric Association. Practice guidelines for the assessment and treatment of suicidal behaviors. Psychiatry online. Available at: http://www.psychiatryonline.com/popup.aspx?aID=56178. Accessed October 20, 2011.
23. Figueroa-Ramos MI, Arroyo-Novoa CM, Lee KA, et al. Sleep and delirium in ICU patients: a review of mechanisms and manifestations. Intensive Care Med 2009;35(5):781–95.
24. Weinhouse GL, Schwab RJ, Watson PL, et al. Bench to bedside review: delirium in ICU patients—importance of sleep deprivation. Crit Care 2009;13(6):234.
25. Tembo AC, Parker V. Factors that impact on sleep in intensive care patients. Intensive Crit Care Nurs 2009;25(6):314–22.
26. Reich M, Rohn R, Lefevre D. Surgical intensive care unit (ICU) delirium: a "psychosomatic" problem? Palliat Support Care 2010;8(2):221–5.
27. Moller MD. State of the science of schizophrenia—what we know and what we don't. In: Abstracts of the 25th APNA Annual Conference. Anaheim, CA, 2011.
28. American Psychiatric Association. Practice guidelines for the assessment and treatment of schizophrenia. Psychiatry online. Available at: http://psychiatryonline.org/content.aspx?bookid=28&sectionid=1665359#46675. Accessed October 22, 2011.
29. Benton T, Staab J, Evans DL. Medical co-morbidity in depressive disorders. Ann Clin Psychiatry 2007;19(4):289–303.
30. Evans DL, Charney DS, Lewis L, et al. Mood disorders in the medically ill: scientific review and recommendations. Biol Psychiatry 2005;58(3):175–89.
31. Bour A, Rasquin S, Aben I, et al. The symptomatology of post-stroke depression: comparison of stroke and myocardial infarction patients. Int J Geriatr Psychiatry 2009;24(10):1134–42.
32. Scherrer JF, Chrusciel T, Zeringue A, et al. Anxiety disorders increase risk for incident myocardial infarction in depressed and nondepressed Veterans Administration patients. Am Heart J 2010;159(5):772–9.
33. Jakobsen AH, Foldager L, Parker G, et al. Quantifying links between acute myocardial infarction and depression, anxiety and schizophrenia using case registry databases. J Affect Disord 2008;109(1-2):177–81.
34. Zalihic A, Markotic V, Mabic M, et al. Differences in quality of life after stroke and myocardial infarction. Psychiatria Danubina 2010;22(2):241–8.
35. Lett HS, Blumenthal JA, Babyak MA, et al. Dimensions of social support and depression in patients at increased psychosocial risk recovering from myocardial infarction. Int J Behav Med 2009;16(3):248–58.

36. Huffman JC, Smith FA, Blais MA, et al. Pre-existing major depression predicts in-hospital cardiac complications after acute myocardial infarction. Psychosomatics 2008;49(4):309–16.
37. Dickens C, McGowan L, Percival C, et al. New onset depression following myocardial infarction predicts cardiac mortality. Psychosom Med 2008;70(4):450–5.
38. Moser DK, Dracup K, Evangelista LS, et al. Comparison of prevalence of symptoms of depression, anxiety, and hostility in elderly patients with heart failure, myocardial infarction, and a coronary bypass graft. Heart Lung 2010;39(5):378–85.
39. Hofhuis JG, Spronk PE, van Stel HF, et al. Experiences of critically ill patients in the ICU. Intensive Crit Care Nurs 2008;24(5):300–13.
40. Cutshall SM, Wentworth LJ, Engen D, et al. Effect of massage therapy on pain, anxiety, and tension in cardiac surgical patients: a pilot study. Complement Ther Clin Pract 2010;16(2):92–5.
41. Bauer BA, Cutshall SM, Wentworth LJ, et al. Effect of massage therapy on pain, anxiety, and tension after cardiac surgery: a randomized study. Complement Ther Clin Pract 2010;16(2):70–5.
42. Brodsky-Israeli M, DeKeyser Ganz F. Risk factors associated with transfer anxiety among patients transferring from the intensive care unit to the ward. J Adv Nurs 2011;67(3):510–8.
43. Vogelzangs H, Seldenrijk A, Beekman AT, et al. Cardiovascular disease in persons with depressive and anxiety disorders. J Affect Disord 2010;125(1–3):241–8.
44. Abu Ruz ME, Lennie TA, Moser DK. Effects of beta-blockers and anxiety on complication rates after acute myocardial infarction. Am J Crit Care 2011;20(1):67–73.
45. Roest AM, Martens EJ, Denollet J, et al. Prognostic association of anxiety post myocardial infarction with mortality and new cardiac events: a meta-analysis. Psychosom Med 2010;72:563–9.
46. Grewal K, Gravely-Witte S, Stewart DE, et al. A simultaneous test of the relationship between identified psychosocial risk factors and recurrent events in coronary artery disease patients. Anxiety Stress Coping 2011;24(4):463–75.
47. Martens EJ, Nyklicek I, Szabo BM, et al. Depression and anxiety as predictors of heart rate variability after myocardial infarction. Psychol Med 2008;38(3):375–83.
48. Kuhl EA, Fauerbach JA, Bush DE, et al. Relation of anxiety and adherence to risk-reducing recommendations following myocardial infarction. Am J Cardiol 2009; 103(12):1629–34.
49. Chung MC, Berger Z, Rudd H. Coping with posttraumatic stress disorder and comorbidity after myocardial infarction. Comp Psychiatry 2008;49(1):55–64.
50. Ayers S, Copland C, Dunmore E. A preliminary study of negative appraisals and dysfunctional coping associated with post-traumatic stress disorder symptoms following myocardial infarction. Br J Health Psychol 2009;14(Pt 3):459–71.
51. Redhead AP, Turkington D, Rao S, et al. Psychopathology in postinfarction patients implanted with cardioverter-defibrillators for secondary prevention: a cross-sectional, case-controlled study. J Psychosom Res 2010;69(6):555–63.
52. Johansson I, Karlson BW, Grankvist G, et al. Disturbed sleep, fatigue, anxiety and depression in myocardial infarction patients. Eur J Cardiovasc Nurs 2010;9(3): 175–80.
53. Friese RS. Sleep and recovery from critical illness and injury: a review of theory, current practice, and future directions. Crit Care Med 2008;36(3):697–705.
54. Hardin KA. Sleep in the ICU: potential mechanisms and clinical implications. Chest 2009;136(1):284–94.

55. Ethier C, Burry L, Martinez-Motta C, et al. Recall of intensive care unit stay in patients managed with a sedation protocol or a sedation protocol with daily sedative interruption: a pilot study. J Crit Care 2011;26(2):127–32.

56. Weinhouse GL, Watson PL. Sedation and sleep disturbances in the ICU. Crit Care Clin 2009;25(3):539–49, ix.

57. Patel M, Chipman J, Carlin BW, et al. Sleep in the intensive care unit setting. Crit Care Nurs Q 2008;31(4):309–18.

58. Scotto CJ, McClusky C, Spillan S, et al. Earplugs improve patients' subjective experience of sleep in critical care. Nurs Crit Care 2009;14(4):180–4.

59. Kronholm E, Laatikainen T, Peltonen M, et al. Self-reported sleep duration, all-cause mortality, cardiovascular mortality and morbidity in Finland. Sleep Med 2011;12(3): 215–21.

60. Sabanayagam C, Shankar A. Sleep duration and cardiovascular disease: results from the National Health Interview Survey. Sleep 2010;33(8):1037–42.

61. Amagai Y, Ishikawa S, Gotoh T, et al. Sleep duration and incidence of cardiovascular events in a Japanese population: the Jichi Medical School cohort study. J Epidemiol 2010;20(2):106–10.

62. Eguchi K, Pickering TG, Schwartz JE, et al. Short sleep duration as an independent predictor of cardiovascular events in Japanese patients with hypertension. Arch Intern Med 2008;168(20):2225–31.

63. Chandola T, Ferris JE, Perski A, et al. The effect of short sleep duration on coronary heart disease risk is greatest among those with sleep disturbance: a prospective study from the Whitehall II cohort. Sleep 2010;33(6):739–44.

64. McEnany GP. Psychopharmacology of sleep and chronic pain/depression. In: Abstracts of the 25th APNA Annual Conference. Anaheim, CA, 2011.

65. Stahl S. Essential psychopharmacology prescriber's guide. New York: Cambridge University Press; 2009.

66. Mohr W. Paychiatric-mental health nursing: evidence-based concepts, skills, and practices. Philadelphia: Lippincott Williams & Wilkins; 2009.

67. Buvanendran A, Kroin JS. Useful adjuvants for postoperative pain management. Best Pract Res Clin Anesthesiol 2007;21(1):31–49.

68. El-Sakka, A. Erectile dysfunction, depression, and ischemic heart disease: does the existence of one component of this triad necessitate inquiring the other two? J Sex Med 2011;8(4): 937–40.

69. Markeljevic J, Sarac H, Rados M. Tremor, seizures and psychosis as presenting symptoms in a patient with chronic lyme neuroborrelliosis. Coll Antropol 2011; 35(Suppl 1):131–8.

70. Miyaoka T, Furuya M, Kristain L, et al. Yi-Gan scan for treatment of Charles Bonnet syndrome (visual hallucination due to vision loss): an open label study. Clin Neuropharmacol 2011;34(1):24–7.

71. Kleffner I, Weresching H, Schwindt W, et al. Triad of visual, auditory and corticospinal track lesions: a new syndrome in a patient with HIV infection. AIDS 2011;25(5):659–63.

72. Erkinjuntti T. Memory complaints, mild cognitive impairment and dementia. Essential Evidence Plus. 2010. Available at: http://www.Essentialevidenceplus.com/content/ebmg_emb/752. Accessed October 5, 2011.

73. Devlin JW, Roberts RJ, Fong JJ, et al. Efficacy and safety of quetiapine in critically ill patients with delirium: a prospective, multi-center, randomized, double-blind, placebo-controlled pilot study. Crit Care Med 2010;38(2):695–6.

74. Clegg A, Young JB. Which medications to avoid in people at risk for delirium: a systematic review. Age Ageing 2011;40(1):23–9.

75. Hoffman L. ACEP recognizes excited delirium syndrome. Emergency Medicine Now's ACEP Scientific Assembly Edition.
76. O'Mahony R, Murthy L, Akunne A, et al; Guideline Development Group. Synopsis of the National Institute for Health and Clinical Excellence guideline for prevention of delirium. Ann Intern Med 2011;154(11):746–51.
77. Sulkava R. Treatment of memory diseases. Essential Evidence Plus. 2009. Available at: http://www.Essentialevidenceplus.com/content/ebmg_emb/758. Accessed October 5, 2011.
78. Capezuti E, Zwicker D, Mezey M, et al. editors.Evidence-based geriatric nursing protocols for best practice. 3rd edition. New York: Springer.
79. Reichman WE, Cummings JL. Dementia. In: Duthie EH, Katz PR, Malone ML, editors. Principles of geriatrics. New York: Saunders Elsevier; 2007. p. 320–34.
80. Malouf R, Birks J. Donepezil for vascular cognitive impairment. (Cochrane Review). In: The Cochrane Library 2009 Issue 1. Chichester, UK: John Wiley and Sons, Ltd.
81. Capell L, Brocato J. Schizophrenia. Essential Evidence Plus. 2011. Available at: http://www.essentialevidenceplus.com/content/ebmg_ebm/711#s4. Accessed October 18, 2011.
82. Colville G, Kerry S, Pierce J. Children's factual and delirium memories of intensive care. Am J Resp Crit Care Med 2008;177:976–82.
83. Crawford MJ, Thana L, Methuen C, et al. Impact of screening for risk of suicide: randomized controlled trial. Br J Psychiatry 2011;198(5):379–84.
84. Cuijpers P, van Straten A, Smit F, et al. Preventing the onset of depressive disorders: a meta-analytic review of psychological interventions. Am J Psychiatry 2008;165(10): 1272–80.
85. Serfaty MA, Haworth D, Blanchard M, et al. Clinical effectiveness of individual cognitive behavioral therapy for depressed older people in primary care: a randomized controlled trial. Arch Gen Psychiatry 2009;66(12):1332–40.
86. Reynolds CF, Dew MA, Pollack BG, et al. Maintenance treatment of major depression in old age. N Engl J Med 2006;354:1130–8.
87. Van Lieshout RJ, MacQueen GM. Efficacy and acceptability of mood stabilizers in the treatment of acute bipolar depression: systematic review. Br J Psychiatry 2010;196: 266–73.
88. Beynon S, Soares-Weiser K, Woolacott N, et al. Psychosocial interventions for the prevention of relapse in bipolar disorder: systematic review of controlled trials. Br J Psychiatry 2010;192:5–11.
89. Sylvia L, Nierenberg AA, Stange, J, et al. Development of an integrated psychosocial treatment to address the medical burden associated with bipolar disorder. J Psychiatr Pract 2011;17(3):224–30.
90. Vieta E, Locklear J, Gunther O, et al. Treatment options for bipolar depression: a systematic review of randomized controlled trials. J Clin Psychopharmacol 2010; 30(4):579–89.
91. Hirschfeld RM. Guideline Watch: practice guidelines for the treatment of patients with bipolar disorder. Arlington(VA): American Psychiatric Association; 2005.
92. Baldwin D, Woods R, Lawson R, et al. Efficacy of drug treatments for generalized anxiety disorder: systematic review and meta-analysis. Br Med J 2011;342:d1199.
93. Shearer SL. Obsessive compulsive disorder. Essential Evidence. Available at: http://www.essentialevidenceplus.com.libproxy2.umdnj.edu/content/eee/828. Accessed November 3, 2011.
94. Benedek DM, Friedman MJ, Zatzick D, et al. Guideline watch: practice guidelines for the treatment of patients with acute stress disorder and posttraumatic stress disorder. Arlington(VA): American Psychiatric Association; 2009.

95. Buscemi N, Vandermeer B, Hooton PR, et al. Melatonin for the treatment of sleep disorders: evidence report/technology assessment No 108. AHRQ publication no. 05-E0021. Rockville(MD): Agency for Healthcare Research and Quality; 2004.
96. Morin CM, Vallieres A, Guay B, et al. Cognitive behavioral therapy, singly and combined with medication for persistent insomnia: a randomized controlled trial. JAMA 2009;301(19):2005–15.
97. Pollack M, Kinrys G, Krystal A, et al. Eszopiclone coadministered in patients with insomnia and comorbid generalized anxiety disorder. Arch Gen Psychiatry 2008;65: 551–62.
98. Morgenthaler TI, Kapur VK, Brown T, et al. Standards of Practice Committee of the American Academy of Sleep Medicine: practice parameters for the treatment of narcolepsy and other hypersomnias of central origin. Sleep 2007;30(12):705–11.
99. Wigus A. Sleep apnea. Essential Evidence. 2011. Available at: http://www. essentialevidenceplus.com/content/eee/692. Accessed November 3, 2011.

Collaborative Partnerships Between Critical Care and Psychiatry

Mary E. Lough, RN, PhD, CNS, CCRN, CNRN, CCNS[a,b,]*, Anne M. Klevay, RN, MSN, PMHCNS-BC[a]

KEYWORDS
- Critical care • Intensive care • Psychiatry • Collaboration
- Interprofessional • Clinical Nurse Specialist • Nursing

The intensive care unit (ICU) and inpatient psychiatry unit are different clinical worlds that care for critical patient populations. Shared clinical diagnoses co-occur for patients with delirium, alcohol withdrawal syndrome, suicide attempts, and major psychiatric disorders such as schizophrenia, bipolar affective disorder, and major depression.

As health care environments and patient needs become increasingly complex, collaboration between diverse patient care areas is expected to increase.[1,2] Research into the transactional elements of interdisciplinary collaboration can provide a helpful lens with which to view trans-professional collaboration.[3] There is a rich literature on the importance of collaboration for the advanced practice nurse (APN)[4–6] and emerging literature related to the importance of teams in the ICU[7–9] including the role of intradisciplinary and interprofessional collaboration across different clinical specialties.[10] D'Amour's model and typology of collaboration between professionals in health care organizations can be used to analyze interprofessional and interorganizational collaborations within any health care organization.[3,10,11] In this article the determinants of successful collaboration are globally presented using an interprofessional collaboration model. The syntax of this conceptual model provides a scaffold to describe collaborative processes between critical care and psychiatry in one academic medical center.

The authors have nothing to disclose.
[a] Stanford Hospital and Clinics, Stanford, 300 Pasteur Drive, H0105, MC5221 Stanford, CA 94305, USA
[b] Department of Physiological Nursing, School of Nursing, University of California–San Francisco, San Francisco, CA, USA
* Corresponding author. Stanford Hospital and Clinics, Stanford, 300 Pasteur Drive, H0105, MC5221 Stanford, CA 94305.
E-mail address: mlough@stanfordmed.org

Crit Care Nurs Clin N Am 24 (2012) 81–90
doi:10.1016/j.ccell.2012.01.003
0899-5885/12/$ – see front matter © 2012 Elsevier Inc. All rights reserved.

INTERPROFESSIONAL COLLABORATIVE FRAMEWORK

D'Amour's interprofessional collaboration model comprises four dimensions. Two dimensions focus on relationships between individuals and two relate to processes within and between organizations. The four component parts are: (1) Shared Goals and Vision, (2) Internalization, (3) Governance, and (4) Formalization.[3] All components are interdependent, interactive, and responsive to change.

Shared Goals and Vision

Shared goals and vision represents one facet of the interpersonal dimension. The strength of multiprofessional teams comes from the perspectives and contributions that arise from health professionals' diverse educational and clinical backgrounds. Ideally members of a team share a common vision and goals. To contribute to successful collaboration, participants must reflect on their own professional interests and biases. From this reflection, team members can negotiate as a team, to achieve consensual shared goals and vision to promote and achieve patient-centered care.[3]

Internalization

Internalization reflects another facet of the interpersonal dimension. Descriptors that reflect the intent of the internalization dimension include mutuality, interdependence, belonging, goodwill, and trust. This conceptualization differs from the professional internalization of role that occurs during the socialization process inherent in all professional practice.[12] Internalization in this context is orientated toward the appreciation of differing and complementary arenas of professional competence and a willingness to assume responsibilities that foster collaboration.[3]

Governance

Governance represents the organizational dimensions that support collaborative innovation between professionals and organizations promoting change. The specific facets of governance that promote interdisciplinary collaboration and foster innovation are centrality, local leadership, support for innovation, connectivity, formalization tools, and information exchange. Centrality is defined as a strong and active central leadership group that actively promotes consensus. Leadership at the local or unit level is focused on consensual decision making in which all voices are equally heard. Support for innovation requires the involvement of individuals with diverse experiences and expertise with recognition that collaboration may result in new solutions to old or recurring problems. It may require that clinical practice responsibilities and resources be shared differently between professionals. Support for innovation in clinical practice is essential to expose silos, facilitate innovation, sustain change, and promote complementary professional growth. Connectivity addresses the organizational requirement for structured forums where exchange of ideas can occur. Optimally this leads to formation of mutual bonds, and improvements in coordination, in response to changing patient care needs.[3]

Formalization

Formalization is an organizational dimension that clarifies professional practice role expectations and division of responsibilities. In hospitals, bedside nursing professional practices are usually codified through policies, procedures, protocols, and contracts. Physician practices and APN practices are codified through institutional credentialing mechanisms. Expansion of the APN role has the potential to alter traditional roles and boundaries and uncertainty about role expectations may ensue. Positive collaborative relationships are more likely when there is consensus about practice roles, shared responsibilities, and established supportive regulations.[3]

Information exchange is a subfacet of formalization that acknowledges the requirement for an effective information-sharing infrastructure between health care professionals. The use of electronic communication and changing work processes can both benefit and stress established collaborative networks. Thus transfer of knowledge and patient care information between professionals is most successful when trust levels are high and uncertainty is minimized. One example of a positive and successful information exchange between critical care and psychiatry is the summarization of organizational resources for managing challenging and disruptive patient behaviors in critical care and medical-surgical units. The psychiatric nurses developed a resource sheet with the categories of Situation, Resources and Details as shown in **Table 1**.

Collaboration between critical care and psychiatry occurs on many professional fronts: between nurses, physicians, APNs, pharmacists, nurse managers, and psychiatric liaison services. In **Fig. 1**, components of D'Amour's model are used to illustrate collaboration dynamics between critical care and psychiatry within a single academic medical center. The outer circle represents organizational infrastructure; the next circle represents collaborative care delivery for the critically ill patient and his or her family. Because of the emotional demands of the ICU work environment, all clinicians need access to social–emotional support. The innermost circle represents the patient and family as the target of collaborative care delivery. Specific psychiatric support functions that are offered to the critical care and medical–surgical units in our institution are listed in **Table 1**.

COLLABORATIVE EXEMPLARS

Optimally, within an organization, multiple opportunities for collaboration occur between critical care and psychiatry. Four exemplars are presented to highlight a variety of collaborative practices between these two patient care specialties: (1) organizational structures that support collaboration, (2) collaboration between staff nurses, (3) implementation of evidence-based practice by the Clinical Nurse Specialist (CNS), and (4) support of critical care nursing staff in times of crisis describes the consultative services of mental health clinicians.[3] These four exemplars help illustrate the interprofessional collaboration model.

Exemplar 1: Organizational Structures

Clinical Nurse Specialists
Governance structural supports within complex organizations can foster collaboration between different professional specialties. The CNS is an APN with specialty education and certification for a defined patient population.[5,13] In this organization, all CNSs report to a single Director of Education and Practice and meet weekly as a group. The meeting time includes a "round table" so colleagues can hear about their peers' achievements and challenges. In this setting opportunities for synergy naturally arise. This creates opportunities for collaboration between CNSs with expertise in very different areas and is helpful to nurses new to the CNS role, new to the institution, or who lack expertise as a change agent. The CNS reporting structure and meeting mechanism would be captured under the dimensions of internalization, governance, and formalization as a component of organizational infrastructure.

Table 1
Managing disruptive and challenging patient behavior

Situation	Resources	Details
Psychiatric symptoms: • **Suicidal Ideation- Psychiatry Service Consult is required** • Depression • Psychosis, mania, confusion, delirium • Combative/ disruptive behavior due to psychiatric illness • Alcohol or Benzodiazepine withdrawal	**Psychiatry Consult Service** • Psychiatrists, M-F, at _____ • On call psychiatrist, at _____ Evenings/ Nights/and Weekends • Nurse Manager to Nurse Manager consult • Contact Inpatient Psychiatry Coordinator at _____ M-F 8:00 AM–5:00 PM • Psychiatric Clinical Nurse Specialist, nurse to nurse consult	• A Psychiatry Consult is **required** for suicidal ideation and recommended for depression (Administrative Manual policy) • Requires physician order • Contact Primary Team to initiate consult
Nurse to Psychiatric Nurse Consult: • Psychotic symptoms • Assistance with nursing strategies in care plan • Disruptive, manipulative, and challenging behavior , patient or family	**Nursing Peer to Peer** • Nursing Managers/Clinical Nurse Specialist • RN Peer-to-Peer telephone consult • Expert psychiatric nurses available for telephone nursing consult, call inpatient units • Nursing Supervisors	**Contact** • Nurse Manager in Psychiatry at _____ • Assistant Nurse Managers in Psychiatry at _____ • Psychiatric Clinical Nurse Specialist at _____ • Call Acute Psychiatry Unit at _____ • Call Medical Psychiatry Unit at _____ • Psychiatric Social Worker is available at _____
Delirium: Acute change or fluctuation in mental status with: inattention, disorganized thinking and/or altered level of consciousness.	**Geriatric Health Services** Contact Geriatric Nurse Practitioner at _____ **Psychiatric Consult Service** Contact Inpatient Psychiatric Coordinator at _____ Mon–Friday or on- call psychiatrist at _____ Evenings/Nights/ Week-ends	• Conduct CAM or CAM- ICU • For 65 years and older, page Geriatric Nurse Practitioner at _____ • For under 65 years, contact Psychiatric Consult Service at _____
Aging Adult Care: Inpatient support for older adult patients & families at risk for care non- adherence after discharge.	**Aging Adult Services** • Program Director at _____ • Nurse Case Managers at _____	• Aging Adult Services works with primary team • Offers consultation, resources, dementia management, coordination of services and follow-up home visits.

Threatening behavior:
- Verbal abuse
- Threatening or violent behavior from Patient/Family (single event, ongoing or escalating behavior)

Call Security for Potentially Assaultive Person
- Call Nursing Supervisor

Call Security at _____
- Security can come to be a "presence" and stay on the unit with the Patient/Family and make frequent rounds in addition to intervening in hostile situations.

Possible illicit drug use:
- Patient may be self-medicating

Security:
- Can perform a room search looking for drugs/dangerous items

Call Security at _____
- Requires physician order, notify physician
- Notify Nursing Supervisor
- Notify Risk Management (done by supervisor)

Customer Service issues:
- Long wait time
- Noisy/difficult roommate situation
- Patient had a difficult experience during hospital stay
- Disgruntled, angry, frustrated, verbally challenging Patient /Family (for single event, ongoing or escalating behavior)

Guest Services
- Concierge Services
- Hospital Information
- Interpreter Services
- Spiritual Care team
- Massage Therapy
- Hospital Musicians
- Smoking Cessation Program

Call Guest Services at _____
- A Guest Services staff person is physically present in hospital: Monday–Friday, 7 AM – 7 PM (On-call person will come to hospital for urgent need)

Conflict between Patient and Family
- Interference with the provision of care

Develop written behavioral
- Contract between Patient / Family and treatment team providers.
- Contact Social worker to facilitate care conference with family

- Work with primary team to develop a contract for treatment
- Use united multi-disciplinary treatment team.

Abbreviations: CAM, Confusion Assessment Method; CAM-ICU, Confusion Assessment Method for the Intensive Care Unit.

This document can be used as a template to formalize contact information and resource sharing between the intensive care unit and psychiatry; Blank spaces are normally filled with contact information such as phone numbers or pager numbers.

Adapted from Managing Disruptive and Challenging Behavior. Psychiatry Resource Nurse project at Stanford Hospital and Clinics, Stanford, CA; with permission.

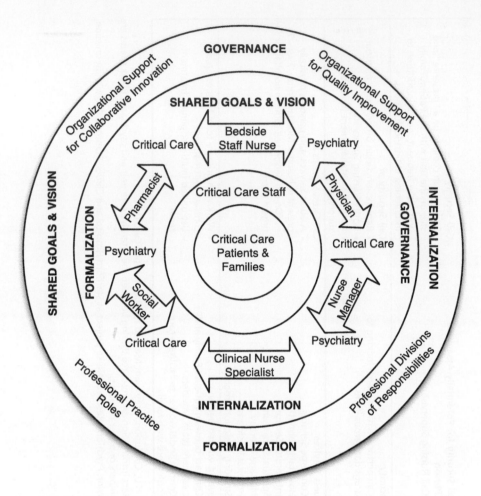

Fig. 1. Interprofessional collaboration between critical care and psychiatry. Core components from D'Amour's Interprofessional Collaboration Model illustrate trans-professional dynamics between critical care and psychiatry within a single academic medical center. The core collaboration components are: Shared Goals and Vision; Internalization; Governance; and Formalization. Moving from the outside circle toward the center: The outer circle represents the organizational infrastructure; the next circle represents interprofessional collaborative roles; the third circle represents critical care staff (any profession) as potentially needing emotional or crisis support as a consequence of the emotionally intense critical care environment; and the central circle emphasizes that the primary collaborative focus is to support the critically ill patient and their family.

Quality Improvement Taskforces

Patient-centered practice changes that traverse disciplines and departments are spearheaded through multiprofessional hospital quality improvement (QI) taskforces. All QI taskforces have CNS members. Multiprofessional QI team work processes can be highly successful or fraught with challenges. It is important that all members perceive the QI taskforce goals as relevant to patient-centered care in their specialty areas. The organizational QI process offers the opportunity to implement evidence-based clinical processes, improve patient care, and support interprofessional collaboration.

Shared Governance

An interdisciplinary shared governance model provides optimal opportunities for transactional professional collaboration using a networked council structure.[14] Core councils are focused on clinical practice, education, research, quality improvement, professional practice, and information technology. Staff nurse involvement is integral to the process. The shared governance structure promotes discussion on patient care issues across patient populations. It is used to disseminate new information, standardize patient care procedures, and implement evidence-based practice innovations. Shared governance as an organizational structure epitomizes all components of interprofessional collaboration, provided membership includes participants of all professions.

Organizations vary in their support for trans-professional collaboration. Absence of such a structure does not mean that collaboration cannot occur. In our experience, professionals with like-minded synergy do find each other in small organizations. In large organizations this may be more difficult and can lead to an isolated practice. We recognize that hospitals differ. Some may not have CNS experts to promote organizational change or lack a synchronized QI process or a shared governance structure. In hospitals without these institutional supports, collaboration still occurs but often on a more informal basis.

Exemplar 2: Collaboration Between Staff Nurses

Peer-to-peer in this context describes nurse-to-nurse collaboration. The charge nurses on the acute psychiatry unit are available for consultation by telephone and in person on a 24-hour basis. In the ICU, clinical situations arise in which patients' or family members' behaviors are demanding, volatile, and disruptive. Psychiatric nurses are available to come to the ICU to review the patient history, meet with the patient or family, and request psychiatric interventions. The psychiatric nurse's expertise in therapeutic communication, setting limits, and deescalating behavioral crisis situations is shared with the critical care nurse through coaching and role modeling.

The benefits of the nurse-to-nurse consult can be elucidated best by a case example. A 54-year-old woman is admitted to the ICU with respiratory distress following bariatric surgery. The patient is morbidly obese, with a Body Mass Index (BMI) greater than 40. Her psychiatric history includes severe depression and Borderline Personality Disorder. The patient has previously been under psychiatric care but use of her prescribed medications were abruptly stopped at the time of the bariatric surgery. She was admitted to the ICU for acute respiratory failure that required several days of ventilatory support. Following extubation significant mood instability and behavioral issues surfaced. The patient became verbally and physically abusive, with intimidating gestures, cursing, pushing nurses away, and refusing to cooperate with nursing care procedures. The psychiatric nurse came to the patient's bedside daily to provide one-to-one support in the ICU. The patient shares that she has felt "dismissed and shamed" all her life. The psychiatric medication regimen is restarted. Subsequent nursing interventions focus on establishing limits and describing respectful behaviors toward nurses that are expected in the ICU. The patient receives assurance that respectful care will be provided in return. With validation some trust is established. This creates a safe environment for both the ICU nurses and the patient during care interventions. The one-to-one support offered daily by the psychiatric nurse is instrumental in diffusing this patient's anger. This exemplar illustrates the concept of internalization, in which professionals with different skill sets recognize and share unique and complementary competencies to collaboratively improve patient care.[3] This intervention is described as a nursing peer-to-peer consultation in **Table 1**.

Exemplar 3: Evidence-Based Practice

The following exemplar highlights collaboration between CNS colleagues within the structure of an organization-wide QI initiative to address delirium in hospitalized patients. Stakeholders from many professions meet weekly for 6 months. The CNSs develop the nurses' role in the early identification of delirium, so that staff nurses can screen all at-risk patients for delirium daily. The published evidence on delirium screening by nonpsychiatric clinicians is used to select valid and reliable instruments that are applicable across many settings. The Confusion Assessment Method (CAM)[15] is selected for the medical–surgical areas, and the CAM-ICU is selected for the ICU.[16] The education and implementation processes were disseminated via the hospital's shared governance structures. The CAM and CAM-ICU are integrated into the electronic health record to facilitate documentation. Resources in the medical–surgical units focus on patients older than 65 years with the highest risk of delirium.[15] A Geriatric Nurse Practitioner position is created to support early identification and management of delirium in the medical–surgical units. The critical care literature does not support an exclusive focus on patients older than 65 years of age, even though older adults are recognized as a high-risk group; consequently all ICU patients are screened for delirium. On a macro level, this exemplar highlights several dimensions of trans-professional collaborative practice: the shared goal and vision of a united multiprofessional team, the governance support for coordinated widespread change and education, and formalization or development of protocols to support new screening procedures and documentation methods across the hospital.[3] On a micro level, this opportunity allowed the two authors to develop a strong collaborative partnership.

Exemplar 4: Support of Critical Care Nursing Staff

The CNS and nurse manager from psychiatry provide support and consultation directly to the ICU staff nurses. An exemplar of supportive consultation originated with the death of a teenage patient in the ICU. Many nurses identify and become close to the young patient and his family during his protracted critical illness. The sudden, although not unexpected, death of the young patient mirrors personal losses in the lives of several staff nurses. Coincidentally, four ICU nurses had recently lost a son to illness or suicide. The cumulative effects of loss and hopelessness on the nursing staff were profoundly felt. The psychiatric CNS and an ICU staff nurse organize a "mourning breakfast" during which natural feelings of loss and grief are richly shared. The nurses affirm their life-long relationships in supporting each other through friendship, pregnancies, launching families, and loss. The CNS facilitates a supportive group to create an atmosphere of warmth, acceptance, and true empathy of lives shared. The nurses openly grieve over the loss of their sons and the young patient. The parallels reveal appreciation of the universality of their experiences and the life meanings they share. Offering a healing presence within a safe space allows natural grief work to unfold and team connections to tighten.

In D'Amour's model this exemplar illustrates the concept of internalization where there is a deep sense of belonging and individuals know each other personally and professionally. Trust in each other is an essential component. There is a strong history of collaboration between ICU and psychiatry. Psychiatric nurses in many roles offer consultation and support to both ICU patients and to ICU nurses.

SYNERGISM

True collaboration occurs when there is a mutually complementary learning process so that synergism develops.[3] Collaboration represents a synergism of skills and professional experiences that produces a whole that is greater than the sum of its parts. Openness to new ideas and a willingness to entertain new perspectives are essential. In a partnership, if one individual has all the knowledge and the other is learning, it is not really a collaborative partnership; it is a mentoring or teacher–student relationship. Successful collaborators both learn and both show-up with open curiosity and the intention to seek fresh perspectives.

Collaboration builds on mutual respect and a high degree of trust. It is probably self evident, but trust once lost is hard to regain. Primary elements that promote trust include the ability to speak truthfully to the shared vision, to have a willingness to "own" and be responsible for a section of the work, to complete that section, communicate unexpected roadblocks, commit to timelines, and still share the results openly. True collaboration leaves no room for territoriality or selective ownership. Because this does not happen in every professional relationship the obvious question is: Can it be developed? Sometimes existing professional relationships have a history of misunderstandings that appear insurmountable. In an ever-changing institutional environment, one strategy for rebuilding trust is to participate in a project with shared goals and vision.

A shared focus on patient outcomes brings out the best in working relationships. Helpful interpersonal skills that further the work of the group and promote collaboration include respecting each person's contribution, not externalizing blame, expressing appreciation, and remaining open to potentially different viewpoints. Acknowledge that overpersonalizing is a sign of stress. Remain optimistic and hopeful with the glass more than half-full.[17] It is helpful to check in with each other to see how the working relationship is going and if either can adjust his or her interactions to promote collegiality.

SUMMARY

The model of collaboration developed by D'Amour and associates can be used to analyze components of collaboration within organizations as shown in **Fig. 1**. The model covers both interprofessional and interorganizational components of collaboration.[3,10,11] A strong supportive organizational infrastructure is the powerful force that sustains successful collaboration between critical care and psychiatry. Professionals' recognition that we have complementary, nonoverlapping clinical skills with recognizance of shared and overlapping populations is vital. The beauty of collaboration is the appreciation of the full value of each participant's unique contribution and diversity. When there are multiple opportunities for collaboration, everyone benefits, especially the critical care patient.

REFERENCES

1. Interprofessional Education Collaborative Expert Panel. Core competencies for interprofessional collaborative practice: report of an expert panel. Washington, DC: Interprofessional Education Collaborative; 2011.
2. Institute of Medicine. The future of nursing: leading change, advancing health. Washington, DC: National Academies Press; 2011.

3. D'Amour D, Goulet L, Labadie JF, et al. A model and typology of collaboration between professionals in healthcare organizations. BMC Health Serv Res 2008;8: 188.

4. Kleinpell RM, Faut-Callahan M, Lauer K, et al. Collaborative practice in advanced practice nursing in acute care. Crit Care Nurs Clin North Am 2002;14(3):307–13.

5. Hanson CM, Spross JA. Collaboration. In: Hamric AB, Spross JA, Hanson CM, editors. Advanced practice nursing: an integrative approach. 4th edition. Saunders Elsevier; 2009. p. 283–314.

6. McNamara S, Lepage K, Boileau J. Bridging the gap: interprofessional collaboration between nurse practitioner and clinical nurse specialist. Clin Nurse Spec 2011;25(1): 33–40.

7. Manthous C, Nembhard IM, Hollingshead AB. Building effective critical care teams. Crit Care 2011;15(4):307.

8. Berlin JM. Synchronous work: myth or reality? A critical study of teams in health and medical care. J Eval Clin Pract 2010;16(6):1314–21.

9. Reinke LF, Hammer B. The role of interprofessional collaboration in creating and supporting health care reform. Am J Respir Crit Care Medicine 2011;184(8):863–4.

10. D'Amour D, Oandasan I. Interprofessionality as the field of interprofessional practice and interprofessional education: an emerging concept. J Interprof Care 2005; 19(Suppl 1):8–20.

11. D'Amour D, Ferrada-Videla M, San Martin Rodriguez L, et al. The conceptual basis for interprofessional collaboration: core concepts and theoretical frameworks. J Interprof Care 2005;19(Suppl 1):116–31.

12. Clark PG. Values in health care professional socialization: implications for geriatric education in interdisciplinary teamwork. Gerontologist 1997;37(4):441–51.

13. Muller A, McCauley K, Harrington P, et al. Evidence-based practice implementation strategy: the central role of the clinical nurse specialist. Nurs Adm Q 2011; 35(2):140–51.

14. Porter-O'Grady T, Parker M, Hawkins M. Interdisciplinary shared governance: a model for integrated professional practice. In: Porter-O'Grady T, editor. Interdisciplinary shared governance: integrating practice, transforming healthcare. 2nd edition. Sudbury (MA): Jones & Bartlett; 2009: 39–74.

15. Inouye SK, Bogardus ST Jr, Charpentier PA, et al. A multicomponent intervention to prevent delirium in hospitalized older patients. N Engl J Med 1999;340(9):669–76.

16. Ely EW, Inouye SK, Bernard GR, et al. Delirium in mechanically ventilated patients: validity and reliability of the confusion assessment method for the intensive care unit (CAM-ICU). JAMA 2001;286(21):2703–10.

17. Marchionni C, Richer MC. Using appreciative inquiry to promote evidence-based practice in nursing: the glass is more than half full. Nurs Leadersh [Tor Ont] 2007; 20(3):86–97.

How Professional Nurses Working in Hospital Environments Experience Moral Distress: A Systematic Review

Dolores M. Huffman, RN, PhD*, Leslie Rittenmeyer, RN, PsyD, CNE

KEYWORDS
- Moral distress • Ethical distress • Moral stress
- Hospital environments

More than 5 million patients with a myriad of challenging illnesses and related health problems are admitted annually to intensive care units (ICUs) in the United States.[1] Caring for these fragile and critically ill patients are the 503,124 critical care nurses employed by hospitals throughout the United States, accounting for an estimated 37% of the total hospital workforce.[2] According to the American Association of Critical-Care Nurses (AACN), critical care nurses work in a nursing specialty that deals specifically with human responses to life-threatening problems and whose responsibility is to ensure that their patients receive optimal care.[2] For some critical care nurses, striving to provide the best possible care for their acutely ill patients amidst an intense, often chaotic and demanding environment, moral distress comes to the forefront and may serve to compromise the patient care they value.

The AACN has addressed concerns regarding moral distress through the creation of a framework to serve as a guide when nurses encounter moral distress. In their document "The 4 A's to Rise Above Moral Distress" nurses are challenged to ask, act, affirm, and assess when confronting issues related to moral distress.[3] The focuses of this paper are on assisting critical care nurses to provide optimal care to their patients and families and use moral distress as a catalyst to create positive changes in their work environment. Further, the AACN in 2008 recognized the seriousness of moral distress in nursing and developed a public policy statement to counteract the convincing evidence that moral distress has a negative impact on the health care environment and retention of nurses in the discipline.[4] The AACN states, "Moral distress is a critical, frequently ignored, problem in healthcare work environments.

School of Nursing, Purdue University Calumet, 2200 169th Street, Hammond, IN 46323, USA
* Corresponding author.
E-mail address: huffman@purduecal.edu

Crit Care Nurs Clin N Am 24 (2012) 91–100
doi:10.1016/j.ccell.2012.01.004
0899-5885/12/$ – see front matter © 2012 Elsevier Inc. All rights reserved.

Unaddressed, it restricts nurses' ability to provide optimal patient care and to find job satisfaction. AACN asserts that every nurse and every employer are responsible for implementing programs to address and mitigate the harmful effects of moral distress in the pursuit of creating a healthy work environment."[4(p1)]

BACKGROUND

Jameton, who first conceptualized moral distress, described it as arising when one knows the right thing to do, but institutional constraints make it nearly impossible to pursue the right course of action.[5] Wilkinson added to Jameton's work and defined moral distress as "the psychological disequilibrium and negative feeling state experienced when a person makes a moral decision but does not follow through by performing the moral behavior indicated by that decision."[6(p16)] In a position statement on moral distress, The American Association of Colleges of Nursing (AACN) described it as occurring when nurses recognize the appropriate action to take, but are unable to act upon it, and further, act in a manner contrary to their personal and professional values, therefore undermining integrity and authenticity.[7] The AACN further identified moral distress as a significant professional problem affecting the physical and emotional health of nurses and impacting quality, quantity, and cost of nursing care.[7] The Canadian Nurses Association (CNA), in a paper entitled "Ethical Distress in Health Care Environments," differentiates between an ethical/moral dilemma and ethical/moral distress. The CNA states that ethical/moral dilemmas "are situations arising when equally compelling ethical reasons both for and against a particular course of action are recognized and a decision must be made . . . ."[8(p3)] Ethical/moral distress occurs when a decision is made regarding what one believes to be the right course of action, but barriers prevent the nurse from carrying out or completing the action."[8(p3)]

Many researchers have identified the deleterious effects of ethical/moral distress.[9–12] Others, such as Kalvermark and colleagues, recognize that the complexities of health care make ethical dilemmas and moral distress inevitable. In the conclusion of their study, the authors suggested that organizations must provide better support, resources, and structures to prevent moral distress.[13] Hefferman and Heilig contended that feelings of powerlessness regarding treatment decisions, high-intensity medical environments, lack of authority, and high responsibility create a recipe for feelings of futility and moral distress.[14] This is supported by Elpern and coworkers, who studied moral distress among staff nurses in a medical ICU and found that critical care nurses are often faced with situations that are associated with high levels of moral distress, which adversely affect job satisfaction, retention, psychological and physical well-being, self-image, and spirituality.[15] In another study, the effects of moral distress were documented as early as 2 years after graduation. Brighid found that relatively new graduates experienced feelings of moral distress as a consequence of believing that they were not living up to their moral convictions and attempting to preserve their moral integrity.[16] In a study that compared nurse–physician perspectives of moral distress and moral climate in the care of dying patients in ICUs, Hamric and Blackhall found that registered nurses experienced more moral distress than did physicians.[17] Corley's study on moral distress of critical care nurses found that of 111 critical care nurses, 12% vacated a nursing position based on their experience of moral distress. In addition, the nurses perceived their ethical environment as more negative and were more critical of the quality of care provided.[18] In their study of moral distress, compassion fatigue, and perceptions about medication errors in certified critical care nurses, Maiden and colleagues found that nurses who experience higher compassion fatigue have higher moral distress. In addition, the researchers suggested that moral distress is a contributing factor requiring further study as it relates to medication errors.[19]

REVIEW OBJECTIVE

The overall objective of this systematic review was to appraise and synthesize the best available evidence on how professional nurses working in hospital environments experience ethical/moral distress. The context was professional nurses experiencing ethical/moral distress as a result of their patient care responsibilities.

METHODOLOGY
Criteria for Considering Studies for this Review

Types of studies
The authors considered qualitative evidence that illuminated the experience of moral distress of professional nurses including, but not limited to, phenomenology, ethnography, grounded theory, hermeneutics, participatory action research, and critical theory. Studies from 1995 to 2008 were included in this review.

Types of participants
This review considered studies whose participants were professional nurses, working in hospital environments and who experienced ethical/moral distress. Experience must have been reported by the nurses themselves.

Phenomena of interest
Studies were included if the focus of the study was a description of the participant's own experience with ethical/moral distress and that experience took place in a hospital environment. The context was professional nurses experiencing ethical/moral distress as a result of their patient care responsibilities.

Types of outcome measures
Outcomes of interest were those that represented the voices of the participants as they related their own experiences of ethical moral distress. Outcomes included, but were not limited to, stress reactions, psychological reactions, feelings of powerlessness, a desire to leave the profession, a perceived lack of administrative support, the stress of being in the role of patient advocate, time/staffing constraints, the devaluing of patient wishes, futile care, unnecessary patient pain and suffering, and perceived employment risk when voicing concerns.

Search Strategy

The comprehensive search strategy aimed to find both published and unpublished studies (**Fig. 1**). The search was limited to English-language reports from 1995 to 2008. A three-step search strategy was utilized in each component of the review. An initial limited search of MEDLINE and Cumulative Index to Nursing and Allied Health Literature (CINAHL) was undertaken followed by analysis of the text words contained in the Joanna Briggs Institute (JBI) Library of Systematic Reviews title and abstract, and the index terms used to describe the article. A second search using all identified keywords and index terms was then undertaken across all included databases. Third, the reference list of identified reports and articles was hand searched for additional studies.
   The databases that were searched include:

   BioMed Central
   CINAHL

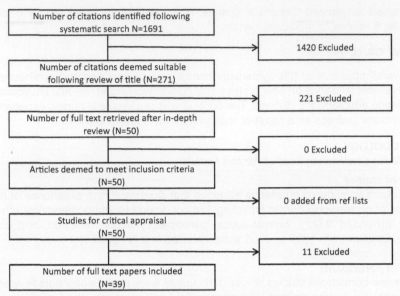

Fig. 1.   Search strategies for published and unpublished studies.

Conference Proceedings Current Contents
EBSCOHost Health Source: Nursing/Academic Edition Elsevier Science Direct EMBASE
Institute for Health & Social Care Research (IHSCR)
MEDLINE
New York Academy of Medicine Grey Literature Report
Nursescribe
Proquest Digital Dissertations
PsycINFO
Reference lists of identified studies and review papers
Science Direct
SCOPUS
Sociological Abstracts
TRIP.

Initial keywords used included moral distress, ethical distress, moral concerns, moral decision*, ethical decision*, ethics, morality.* A technique of Boolean Logic and serves as a strategy for on-line library searching. (ie, It helps to identify moral decisions, moral decision-making etc).

Assessment of Methodological Quality

Research papers selected for appraisal were assessed by the two authors for methodologic quality before inclusion. The review used standardized critical appraisal instruments from the Joanna Briggs Institute, specifically the Qualitative Assessment and Review Instrument (QARI). The two authors were experienced nurses and academics as well as qualitative researchers. Consultation with a third reviewer to resolve any disagreements was available as a contingency but was not required. A cutoff point of 6 out of the 10 questions answered with a "yes" was established as a general guideline by the authors. QARI is the software component of the SUMARI suite that supports the synthesis of qualitative research evidence. QARI facilitates the reviewer's assessment of the congruency between philosophical perspective and research methodology, research question and methods, data collection and methods analysis and interpretation, participants' voices, and ethical conduct in the conduction of research. See **Fig. 1** for search results.

Data Collection/Extraction

Data were extracted from papers included in the review using the standardized data extraction tool from QARI. Data extracted from interpretive and critical research included specific details about the type of text, representation, position, setting, geographical and cultural information, the logic of the argument, and the type of data analysis used to determine conclusions and credibility of evidence. Each finding that was extracted was assigned a level of credibility.

Data Synthesis

Data were synthesized using QARI to pool the findings. This process included the synthesis of findings to generate a set of statements that represent that aggregation through assembling the findings (Level 1 findings) rated according to their quality and categorizing those findings on the basis of similarity of meaning (Level 2 findings). Those categories were then subjected to a meta-synthesis to produce a single comprehensive set of synthesized findings (Level 3 findings) that could be used for evidence-based practice. This review produced 101 findings that were aggregated into 11 categories, resulting in 4 synthesized findings.

RESULTS
Methodologic Quality

Of the 50 critically appraised studies, 11 were excluded, but most for reasons other than methodologic quality. Some of the studies included participants from more than one discipline and it was difficult to identify the voices of the professional nurses; in other studies it was not possible to identify the context of the research and in others moral distress was measured using a tool.

Results of the Meta-Aggregate of Qualitative Research Findings

Meta-synthesis of studies included in the review generated four synthesized findings. These synthesized findings were derived from 102 study findings that were subsequently aggregated into 11 categories. The findings indicated that many nurses express moral distress through biopsychosocial responses such as anger, depression, and stress reactions. There is also a tendency by nurses who experience moral distress to withdraw emotionally from patients. Moral distress was also experienced when nurses felt powerless to implement change or influence decision making The categories of Biopsychosocial Responses, Emotional Withdrawal, and Powerlessness led to the first synthesis finding of Human Reactivity, defined as the experience of moral distress that causes nurses to respond with a myriad of reactions including anger, loneliness, depression, guilt, anxiety, feelings of powerlessness, and emotional withdrawal, all of which lead to related physical symptomatology.

The findings also indicated that when nurses experience moral distress over time there are frequently deleterious effects on the health care system, such as nurses leaving the institution, leaving the profession, or moving to less stressful jobs. Health care system constraints such as limited finances, weak policies, and poor staffing patterns significantly contribute to the experience of moral distress. In addition, moral distress was experienced when nurses advocated for patients and their voices were not acknowledged. The categories of Adverse Effects to the System, Health Care Constraints, and Patient Advocacy created the second synthesis finding of Institutional Culpability, defined as the experience of moral distress when nurses felt the need to advocate for patients' well-being while coping with institutional constraints. The deleterious effect was often nurses leaving the institution or profession.

Feelings of moral distress were experienced when nurses saw others devaluing the wishes of patients and families. Similar feelings were experienced when nurses perceived that patients were suffering as a result of their treatment or lack of it. This was also true when nurses observed patients being subjected to treatments that they perceived as futile. The categories of Devaluing Patient Wishes, Patient Suffering, and Futile Care created the third synthesis finding of Patient Pain and Suffering. Patient Pain and Suffering is defined as the experience of moral distress when nurses perceive that patients are receiving futile care and their wishes are ignored by physicians, institutions, or families. The perception of patient suffering as result of medical decisions was extremely distressful.

Lastly, moral distress was experienced when there were conflicting professional goals and values that were inconsistent with the science and values inherent in the discipline of nursing. Moral distress was also felt when physicians and others failed to include the nurse as a valuable member of the health care team, capable of contributing to and influencing treatment goals. The categories of Conflicting Professional Goals and Values, and Unequal Authority led to the fourth synthesis finding of Unequal Hierarchies, defined as the experience of moral distress when nurses perceived that physicians and others devalued nursing expertise and displayed a lack of recognition of nursing authority when there was a difference in professional goals and values. The fact that physician authority is assumed and seldom questioned contributes to the perception of inequality.

DISCUSSION

The purpose of this systematic review was to examine the best available evidence on the ways in which professional nurses, working in hospital environments, experience ethical/moral distress. To address this question, qualitative studies using a myriad of methodologies such as phenomenology, descriptive/exploratory, participatory action research, grounded theory, and hermeneutics were identified. Using the JBI-QARI tools from the Joanna Briggs Institute, the authors critically (**Fig. 2**) appraised 50 research reports and retained 39 for data extraction. A total of 101 findings were extracted and these generated 11 categories. These categories were then analyzed to identify four syntheses:

1. Human Reactivity: Nurses who experience moral distress respond with a myriad of biological, psychological, and stress reactions.
2. Institutional Culpability: Moral distress is experienced when nurses feel the need to advocate for patients' well-being while coping with institutional constraints.
3. Patient Pain and Suffering: The perception of patient pain and suffering as a result of medical decisions, of which the nurse has little power to influence, contribute to the experience.
4. Unequal Power Hierarchies: Unequal power structures, prevalent in institutions, exacerbate the problem.

Nurses who experience moral distress responded with a myriad of human reactions including anger, loneliness, depression, guilt, anxiety, feeling of powerlessness, and emotional withdrawal. Nurses not only withdrew within themselves but also withdrew

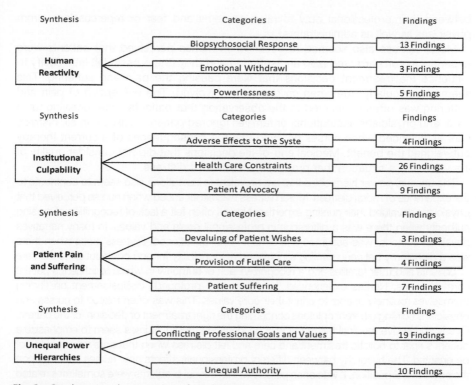

Synthesis	Categories	Findings
Human Reactivity	Biopsychosocial Response	13 Findings
	Emotional Withdrawl	3 Findings
	Powerlessness	5 Findings
Institutional Culpability	Adverse Effects to the Syste	4 Findings
	Health Care Constraints	26 Findings
	Patient Advocacy	9 Findings
Patient Pain and Suffering	Devaluing of Patient Wishes	3 Findings
	Provision of Futile Care	4 Findings
	Patient Suffering	7 Findings
Unequal Power Hierarchies	Conflicting Professional Goals and Values	19 Findings
	Unequal Authority	10 Findings

Fig. 2. Syntheses and categories of qualitative studies.

emotionally from patients. The stress from these reactions often led to related physical symptoms. Examples of biopsychosocial responses were prevalent in the findings. Narratives about feeling sick, stressed, powerless, numb, angry, depressed, and frustrated and anxious were rich. Nurses reported that moral distress produced a variety of strong negative feelings, making the work environment an unpleasant place to be.

The participants' narratives suggest that there is an institutional culpability in contributing to the experience of moral distress. This seemed to be true despite the geographical/cultural context. Moral distress is felt most intensely when nurses feel they need to advocate for patients' well-being while coping with institutional constraints. Experiencing moral distress seemed to heighten nurses' sense of patient advocacy. The deleterious effects of this on the health care system were reported as the desire to work part time, leave the unit, leave the institution, or leave the profession. Job satisfaction/retention seems to be one of the major deleterious effects of nurses experiencing moral distress. The constraints imposed by the institutional system sometimes brought some nurses to believe that they could not practice nursing in accordance with their value system. Unrealistic and unsafe staffing patterns causing increased workloads, and the deleterious effects on patient care were common in the narratives. An inability to have interpersonal relationships with patients was often reported as a frustration. Nurses often felt squeezed between what they know they should do and want to do and institutional constraints that focus only on cost containment. Nurses acutely experienced moral distress when they felt an inability to provide quality of care because of financial constraints and staffing cutbacks. Raising concerns about quality of care, dilemmas, and difficulties were experienced by some nurses as feelings of dissonance between their professional duty to raise concerns and fear of repercussions—from physicians as well as administrators.

Moral distress also seemed to occur when nurses perceived that patients were experiencing unwarranted pain and suffering and they (the nurses) felt little ability to influence the treatment decisions that were causing the pain and suffering. This seemed particularly true when children were involved. The perception of pain and suffering was often connected to the observation that patients were receiving futile care, and physicians, institutions, or families ignored patients' wishes. In all, distress was experienced when nurses believed that the consequences of a current therapy outweighed the benefit. Medical end-of-life decisions that did not consider quality of life were also a situation that produced a climate of distress.

The unequal power hierarchies that are prevalent in institutions also seem to contribute to the experience of moral distress. Moral distress was experienced when nurses perceived that physicians devalued their nursing expertise. Nurses often felt a lack of recognition of nursing authority when there was a difference in professional goals and values. In many narratives physician authority was assumed and almost never questioned. Distress arose when there was a dichotomy between nursing's increased responsibility for and contribution to the care of patients and their families and a recognized lack of authority in which to influence patient care decisions. Nurses experienced "relentless and profound" disillusionment on finding themselves routinely unable to enact their core values. This was often related to nurses and physicians holding different opinions concerning the right treatment or decision for the patient. Overly aggressive medical treatment was an identified theme. Nurses seem to emphasize a patient's right to holistic treatment and care and felt distress when that core value could not be enacted. The hierarchy between different professionals affects how nurses can act upon their own moral position. It was often perceived that ethical problems were sometimes related to nurses' lower position in the hierarchical structure.

SUMMARY

The experience of moral distress for professional nurses working in hospital environments causes a myriad of biological, psychological, and stress-related reactions. There is an institutional culpability in producing an environment where moral distress is experienced. This is particularly true when nurses feel the need to advocate for patients' well-being while coping with institutional constraints. The perception of patient pain and suffering as a result of medical decisions, which the nurse has little power to influence, contributes to the experience. Unequal power structures, prevalent in institutions, exacerbate the problem.

Critical care nurses need to recognize moral distress and its adverse impact on providing optimal patient care. Critical care nurses should make a personal commitment that moral distress will not impact their nursing care and take a leadership role in their units to address this issue with their employing institution and develop strategies to lessen the impact of moral distress. These strategies should be based on the best available evidence such as this systematic review and other relevant appraised works.

Implications for Nursing Practice

From the review and syntheses, several recommendations for practice emerge:

- Institutions need to recognize nursing specialties such as critical care that may be at increased risk for experiencing moral distress.
- Institutions need to consider the implementation of the American Association of Critical-Care Nurses framework addressing moral distress.

- Institutions need to design structures that provide support for nurses who are experiencing feelings of moral distress. These structures need to be genuine, nonjudgmental, and ideally provided by nurses.
- Professional nurses need to have access to the ethics committee of the institution.
- Education programs that teach nurses how to recognize moral distress and the effects it has on the mind and body should be offered and nurses given time to attend.
- Institutions need to provide front line nurses a voice in expressing concerns about health care constraints and invite input on problem solving.
- Institutions need to create an environment of shared respect, acknowledging nurses' contributions and supporting autonomous nursing intervention.
- The nursing value of holistic care needs to be respected by institutions.
- Nurses should not be coerced into violating their own core beliefs about what constitutes good nursing care, especially in their role of patient advocates.

Implications for Research

Several registered nurses experiencing moral distress expressed a desire for an established support system within their employing institution such as easy accessibility to a hospital-based ethics committee, open communications with nurse managers, and established ethical support groups. Further research is needed on the perceived effectiveness of these strategies in addressing the nurses' experience of moral distress and preventing potential nurse burnout.

In addition, further study is warranted on the perceived hierarchal structure of the physician–nurse relationship within the context of the hospital environment. Participants in the included research studies described the inherent "risk" involved in advocating for patients. This risk contributed to their moral distress and was frequently associated with physician decision making that violated the wishes of the patients and required nurses to unwillingly participate in futile care endeavors. An investigation is needed of strategies that provide an equalizing voice for registered nurses and decrease a sense of powerlessness in providing patient-centered care.

REFERENCES

1. Society of Critical Care Medicine. Critical care statistics in the United States. Available at: http://www.siriusgenomics.com/content/technology/CriticalCareStatistics.pdf. Published 2006. Accessed November 12, 2011.
2. American Association of Critical-Care Nurses (AACN). About critical care nursing. Available at: http://www.aacn.org/wd/publishing/content/pressroom/aboutcriticalcarenursing.pcms?pid=1&&menu=practice. Accessed November 11, 2011.
3. American Association of Critical Care Nurses (AACN) from AACN Ethics Work Group. The 4 A's to rise above moral distress. (2004). Available at: http://www.aacn.org/WD/Practice/Docs/4As_to_Rise_Above_Moral_Distress.pdf. Published 2004. Accessed November 11, 2011.
4. American Association of Critical Care Nurses (AACN). Moral distress: AACN public policy position statement. http://www.aacn.org/WD/Practice/Docs/Moral_Distress.pdf. Published August, 2008. Accessed November 11, 2011.
5. Jameton A. Nursing practice: the ethical issues. Englewood Cliffs (NJ): Prentice-Hall; 1984.
6. Wilkinson JM. Moral distress in nursing practice: experience and effect. Nurs Forum 1988;23:16–29.

7. American Association of Colleges of Nursing (AACN). Moral distress. Available at: http://www.aacn.org/aacn/pubpolcy.nsf/vwdoc/pmp. Accessed January 23, 2008.
8. Canadian Nurses Association (CAN). Ethical distress in health care environments. Available at: http://www.cnanurses.ca/can/documents/pdf/publications/ethics_Pract_Ethical_Issues_June_1998_e.pdf. Published June, 1998. Accessed January 23, 2008.
9. Sundin-Huard D, Fahy K. Moral distress, advocacy and burnout. Int J Nurs Pract 1999;5:8–13.
10. Erlin J. Moral distress: a pervasive problem. Orthop Nurs 2001;20:76–80.
11. Fry S, Harvey R, Hurley A, et al. Development of a model of moral distress in military nursing. Nurs Ethics 2003;9:373–87.
12. Gutierrez KM. Critical care nurses' perceptions of and responses to moral distress. Dimens Crit Care Nurs 2005;24:229–41.
13. Kalvemark S, Hoglund A, Hansson M, et al. Living with conflicts—ethical dilemmas and moral distress in the health care system. Soc Sci Med 2003;58:1075–84.
14. Hefferman P, Heilig S. Giving moral distress a voice: ethical concerns among neonatal intensive care unit personnel. Cambridge Quart Healthcare Ethics 1999;8:173–8.
15. Elpern E, Covert B, Kleinpell R. Moral distress of staff nurses in a medical intensive care unit. Am J Crit Care 2005;14:523–30.
16. Brighid K. Preserving moral integrity: a follow up study with new graduate nurses. J Adv Nurs 1998;28:1134–45.
17. Hamric A, Blackhall L. Nurse–physician perspectives on the care of dying patients in intensive care units: collaboration, moral Distress and ethical climate. Crit Care Med 2007;35:422–9.
18. Corley MC. Moral distress of critical care nurses. Am J Crit Care 1995;4:280–5.
19. Maiden J, Georges JM, Connelly CD. Moral distress, compassion fatigue, and perceptions about medication errors in certified critical care nurses. Dimens Crit Care Nurs 2011;30:339–45.

Critical Care Nursing and Delirium Management in the Mentally Ill Client

Yolanda Bone, RN, BSN, CCRN[a],*,
George Byron Smith, DNP, ARNP, GNP-BC[b]

KEYWORDS
- Delirium • Psychosis • Nurse perception

Following a tumultuous intraoperative course involving an initial coronary artery bypass graft and a subsequent return due to hemorrhage, Mr J, 55, is admitted to the cardiac surgical intensive care unit (CSICU). Mr J is successfully extubated and is hemodynamically stable, despite hemoglobin of 8 and a hematocrit of 24. Mr J states he feels weak and "out of sorts." During the nursing admission and assessment process, the nurse learns from Mr J's wife that he has a history of hypertension, coronary artery disease, active smoking, and bipolar disorder. The critical care nurse determines that Mr J stopped taking all of his medications, including his psychotropic medications, two days prior to surgery.

The next day, Mr J is confused and disoriented. He states, "There are bugs all over me!" and is attempting to get out of the bed. The critical care nurse calls the doctor to attain orders for a sedative that she subsequently provides to the client. After this, Mr J calms down; the nurse attributes Mr J's symptoms to his diagnosis of bipolar disorder. "He's probably psychotic and/or manic after everything he has been through, poor guy. He needs to transfer to the psych unit as soon as possible," states the critical care nurse to a colleague. However, is Mr J exhibiting symptoms of psychosis, or are his symptoms related to critical care delirium?

The following case study describes a situation in which a client with multiple health issues is admitted to CSICU following surgery. The client began displaying signs of confusion that the critical care nurse interpreted as being related to his psychiatric illness, thus she ceased assessing causes. There are many reasons for the client to be experiencing confusion. He may be reacting to pain medications or be sleep

The authors have nothing to disclose.
[a] College of Nursing, Critical Care, South University, Tampa Campus, 4401 North Himes Avenue, Tampa, FL 33614, USA
[b] College of Nursing, Psychiatric-Mental Health Nursing, South University, Tampa Campus, 4401 North Himes Avenue, Tampa, FL 33614, USA
* Corresponding author.
E-mail address: ybone@southuniversity.edu

deprived. He may be reacting to his low hemoglobin and hematocrit, or he may be experiencing tobacco withdrawal. In addition, he may be experiencing withdrawal of his psychotropic medications. This client has multifactorial problems that may be causing his confusion and erratic behavior; yet, in this scenario the critical care nurse is attributing it only to his bipolar diagnosis. Is this client demonstrating symptoms of psychosis related to bipolar disorder or is it delirium based on other factors?

DEFINE PSYCHOSIS VERSUS DELIRIUM

Delirium is a common and serious transient cognitive condition in critically ill patients. The prevalence of delirium in intensive care units (ICUs) is high and has been shown to prolong hospitalizations and to increase morbidity and mortality.[1] The word "delirium" is derived from the Latin term *de liro* meaning "deviation from the straight track" or "off the track." The Diagnostic and Statistical Manual of Mental Disorders (DSM-IV) defines delirium as a psychiatric disorder characterized by a disturbance of consciousness with inattention accompanied by a change in cognition or perceptual disturbance that develops in a short period (hours to days) and fluctuates over time.[2]

There are four diagnostic criteria for delirium: (1) altered or disturbance of consciousness with an impaired awareness of the environment and an inability to maintain focused attention, (2) a change in cognition or a perceptual disturbance unaccounted by a preexisting demented state, (3) develops over a short period of time (from hours to days) and fluctuates over the course of the day, and (4) evidence from the history, physical examination, and laboratory findings indicates that the disturbance is caused by the direct physiological consequences of a general medical condition.

Not unlike delirium, psychosis is an exacerbation of symptoms that can increase morbidity and mortality in the critical care patient; however, psychosis generally does not occur as quickly as delirium. In general, critical care nurses are more likely to observe delirium rather than psychosis due to the intensive care unit course of stay. If symptoms arise, critical care nurses should have some sense of identification in order to care for these clients.

Psychosis is a disorderly mental state in which a client has difficulty distinguishing reality from his or her own internal perceptions.[3] Unlike other chronic conditions that can be examined via blood tests and other diagnostic criteria, psychosis manifests itself as an increase in bizarre behavior and/or abnormal language.[4] Symptoms may arise related to stoppage of antipsychotic medication, stressors related to the critical care environment, and complications related to critical illness. Acute psychosis can last from 1 to 4 months; therefore, it is essential that critical care nurses provide an environment in which symptoms may not occur.

NURSE PERCEPTIONS

Critical care nurses are specialized in the assessment and care of persons experiencing life-threatening problems. Critical care nurses work wherever critically ill patients are found—ICUs, pediatric ICUs, neonatal ICUs, cardiac care units, cardiac catheter labs, telemetry units, progressive care units, emergency departments, and recovery rooms. Critical care nurses are adept at determining a change in health status, reacting to that change, and implementing practices to improve outcomes. Yet, critical care nurses, like other nurses outside the realm of mental health, feel inadequately prepared to care for the needs of the individual with a psychiatric diagnosis.

Nursing is the symbiosis of science and compassion. The holistic approach to nursing views an individual as having a balance. Illness causes an imbalance, and nurses address this imbalance wholly. Mental illness is viewed in a different manner. The critical care nurse acknowledges the presence of mental illness; yet, she prioritizes the critical illness at hand and "boxes" the mental illness. "Let's get this guy medically cleared and out of here" is a common care plan for the client who has an exacerbation of psychiatric symptoms following a critical illness. This is a problem. Nurses outside of mental health tend to view a "psych" patient by their psychological needs only, rather than by the whole picture. Why are psychiatric diagnoses viewed upon as the entirety of a person? Other illnesses, such as hypertension or coronary artery disease, do not create patient-labels as does mental health. Holistic practice means the whole client. What causes the critical care nurse to perceive inadequacy to care properly for these clients?

Arnold & Mitchell examined perceptions of acute care nurses caring for clients with mental health illnesses.[5] Themes identified included mental health issues, training and education, and collaborative working.

Mental health issues are related to understanding behavior and symptoms related to varying diagnoses. Mental health disorders are considered a separate illness instead of a component of the health continuum of the individual. Consequently, acute care nurses focus on systemic illnesses such as diabetes and hypertension, and they feel the "behavioral" disease is outside of their realm. This is the similar perception of mental health nurses caring for clients with "physical" illnesses. Mental health nurses are uncomfortable managing the "physical" illnesses, stating it is outside of their realm. In actuality, critical care environments and mental health units should be viewed in similar fashions; meaning that these areas deal with severe exacerbations of health imbalances. A client with a mood disorder having suicidal ideation will be appropriately placed on the mental health unit in order to reduce symptoms and maintain balance. In a similar way, a patient with exacerbation of congestive heart failure will be admitted to the coronary care unit to attain homeostasis. In both care areas, clients with comorbidities will be admitted. The idea for nurses to recognize is the health of a person is complete. One problem is not separate from another. Although acute care facilities separate health problems, a person's health cannot be disconnected.

A way to alleviate the concerns of critical care nurses is through education. Critical care nurses are provided up-to-date information concerning disease processes depending on the unit specialty. For example, in coronary care units, nursing staff will be educated on new procedures and evidence-based practice methods related to myocardial infarction. In addition, in-services concerning new products and new medications will be provided to staff. Providing education snippets on the symptoms of psychosis, mental health issues, and medication modalities may empower critical care nurses. The goal should not be to turn a critical care nurse into a mental health nurse, but rather to provide the nurse with the tools to ensure positive patient outcomes.

Collaborative practice employs sharing of clinical knowledge, providing recommendations for assessment and treatment, and providing professional support. Mental health nurses could provide collaborative support to critical care nurses when a client is displaying mental health symptoms. In addition, recommendations to prevent exacerbation of illness can be a product of this teamwork.

ASSESSMENT AND INTERVENTION

Early assessment and intervention of psychiatric symptoms can alleviate other complications related to the intensive care experience such as delirium. In addition, assessment and intervention of delirium can prevent an exacerbation of psychiatric symptoms. The management of psychiatric problems should not be acted upon following the critical care event. Critical care nurses are skilled assessors of change in health status. It is understood that changes in vital signs alert nurses to intervene and prevent poorer outcomes. This principle can be applied to the client with the comorbidity of a psychiatric diagnosis. An alteration in this balance can affect the client's whole outcome, causing a longer critical care course and increasing mortality risk.

Assessment measures can be implemented with usage of delirium tools such as the Intensive Care Delirium Screening Checklist and the Confusion Assessment Method (CAM) for ICU patients. These tools have been specifically designed to help nurses and other health care professionals identify the presence of delirium. Critical care nurses use sedation tools like the Ramsey Scale; therefore, implementation of a delirium tool is not out of the scope of practice. The key is education. As indicated earlier, critical care nurses are adept at changes in condition; therefore, delirium and psychosis can be noted by these practitioners.

SUMMARY

The critical care environment is an experience of stress for the patient and the practitioner. Turbulence can occur during the critical care course, which can cause exacerbation of chronic conditions. These exacerbations can lead to delirium and/or psychosis. Nursing professionals must be alert to changes in all conditions which increase morbidity and mortality in the critical care patient. Although critical care nurses may feel unable to care for the psychiatric needs of clients with a chronic mental disorder, implementing tools to aid in assessment will empower the nurses.

Truly, the key to viewing all clients is wholly, rather than by diagnosis. Critical care nurses care for clients with many comorbidities and illnesses. Many conditions may be a new experience. Mental disorders should not be viewed as being out of the scope of the critical care nurse. On the contrary, mental disorders are chronic conditions, not unlike diabetes mellitus or congestive heart failure. What the critical care nurse needs is a knowledge base in order to feel more comfortable in caring for these clients. Knowledge is empowerment.

REFERENCES

1. Girard TD, Pandharipande PP, Ely EW. Delirium in the intensive care unit. Crit Care 2008(Suppl 3):S3.
2. American Psychiatric Association (APA). Diagnostic and statistical manual of mental disorders: DSM-IV-TR. Washington, DC: APA; 1994.
3. Vacek JE. Using a conceptual approach with a concept map of psychosis as an exemplar to promote critical thinking. J Nurs Ed 2009;48(1):49–53.
4. Theodoridou C, Bowers L, Brennan G, et al. The measurement of psychotic acuity by nursing staff. J Psychiatr Ment Health Nurs 2009;16:234–41.
5. Arnold M, Mitchell T. Nurses' perceptions of care received by older people with mental health issues in an acute hospital environment. Nurs Older People 2008; 20(10):28–34.

Straddling the Fence: ICU Nurses Advocating for Hospice Care

Deborah Borowske, DNP, MSN, RN, GCNS-BC[a,b,*]

KEYWORDS

• End of life • Hospice • Intensive care unit • Nursing

Every day, nurses in the intensive care unit (ICU) care for critically ill, elderly patients who have not been offered the option of hospice care. With hospice's introduction to the United States in the 1970s, a movement to improve overmedicalization and institutionalization of care for the dying emerged. Despite the steady growth in hospice utilization, many prospective enrollees are not offered the comprehensive comfort care that is a cornerstone of hospice. Many patients are referred late or not at all; more than 60% of adult Americans die without the benefit of hospice care.[1] In addition, of the patients enrolled, more than one third die within 7 days of enrollment.[1] Medicare reports that 11% of beneficiaries spend longer than 7 days in an ICU within the final 6 months of life and of those ICU admissions, only 35% to 50% of all elderly patients survive to discharge.[2]

With a booming geriatric population, ICU nurses face a daily struggle with why they keep doing the same thing, again and again, for chronically ill elderly patients who have little chance of surviving hospitalization or returning to prehospitalization functionality. The ICU nurse feels a duty to follow physician orders, while questioning the futility of aggressive treatments in the face of probable death, or at the minimum, significantly poor quality of life if the patient survives. During the ICU stay, many patients receive mechanical ventilation, artificial nutrition, dialysis, artificial hydration, frequent x-rays, daily laboratory testing, minor procedures, and inadequate pain management. The ICU nurse feels responsible for participating in these ongoing and aggressive therapies, inflicting suffering on elderly patients, while delivering interventions that are not aligned with the patient's ability to recover. The result is moral distress for the ICU nurse participating in care that will ultimately end in a "bad death."[3] A "good death" as defined by the Institute of Medicine as "one that is free

The author has nothing to disclose.
a Department of Community Health, Geriatrics, Hospice and Home Health, Southwest General Health Center, 18697 Bagley Road, Middleburg Heights, OH 44130, USA
b Kent State College of Nursing, Kent State University, Kent, OH, USA
* Department of Hospice, Southwest General Health Center, 18697 Bagley Road, Middleburg Heights, OH 44130.
E-mail address: dborowske@swgeneral.com

Crit Care Nurs Clin N Am 24 (2012) 105–116
doi:10.1016/J.ccell.2012.01.006
0899-5885/12/$ – see front matter © 2012 Elsevier Inc. All rights reserved.

from avoidable distress and suffering for patient, families and caregivers: in general accord with patients' and families' wishes; and reasonably consistent with clinical cultural and ethical standards."[4]

HOSPICE OVERVIEW

Hospice is designed to provide optimal end-of-life (EOL) care for patients with a life-limiting illness and a prognosis of 6 months or less. Customized to the patient's unique needs and wishes, a hallmark of hospice care includes expert medical care, pain and symptom management, and emotional and spiritual support. The emphasis is on caring, not curing, and is usually provided in the patient's place of residence (private home, senior apartment, or assisted living facility), although it can also be provided in a residential hospice facility, hospital, nursing home, or other long-term care facility. Care is patient centered and includes support for the deceased patient's family with bereavement services up to 13 months after death. Family satisfaction surveys report high satisfaction with hospice, along with regret of not beginning hospice sooner during the illness.[5] Patients can be enrolled from any setting into hospice care, including the ICU.

Despite the clear benefits of hospice care and the high percentage of patients in the ICU who meet eligibility for hospice, along with nurses identifying the futility of treatment, studies show that hospice is not always discussed.[6] Why? A number of barriers leading to underutilization and late hospice enrollments have been identified, which lead to the current delays in discussing hospice as an option on the care continuum.

REVIEW OF THE LITERATURE
Patient Barriers

The most prominent barrier for hospice enrollment is the patient's fear of death. Patients often perceive hospice as a last resort for when their death is projected to be days away and they have exhausted all treatment options. The decision to enroll in hospice is extremely difficult within that emotional framework and is heavily influenced by the timing of the referral, their understanding of the trajectory of their illness, their insight into determining what is most important to them as they approach the end of their life, and finally what they are willing to endure to prolong their life.[7-9] Processing these factors is a struggle for most patients, their families, and sometimes their physicians. Even in situations where hospice has been discussed and is being considered, decisions to enroll are postponed while the patient and family engage in multiple hospice information visits, ultimately resulting in delayed enrollment.[10,11]

In the ICU, the majority of patients are unable to make treatment decisions. As a result, families act as decision makers and grapple with the gravity of "giving up" versus "doing everything that can be done." Clinicians are often uninformed as to what the family knows about the current healthcare crisis and the events leading up to the hospitalization. When family is queried about their general knowledge of the components of hospice, studies found most patients and families referred for a hospice information visit knew little about hospice and had substantial education needs.[12-14] They lacked an understanding of the scope of hospice services, from skilled nursing care and symptom management to the comprehensive financial coverage provided under the hospice benefit. Frequently, families were unaware of the palliative care features that would keep their loved one comfortable, manage troublesome symptoms such as air hunger, terminal restlessness, anxiety, and agitation, while simultaneously helping the family to understand and feel prepared for the dying process.[15-20]

Physician Barriers

Physicians fail to discuss the truth about prognosis.[21] Reasons included perceived lack of training, stress, emotional frailty of the patient, fear of negative impact on the patient, uncertainty about prognostication, requests from family to withhold information, and feelings of inadequacy or hopelessness regarding the unavailability of further curative treatment.[22] Huskamp and colleagues[23] found, in a large multiregional study of 1517 patients with stage IV lung cancer, that more than half of the patients did not have any discussion with their physicians about hospice or palliative care, yet died within 6 months of the study. Because the culture of medicine is to cure and prolong life, referral to hospice may be viewed as a medical failure.[24] Referring to hospice accentuates the physicians' perception of failure and they find it difficult to abandon curative measures. Further, the requirement that a physician must certify that the patient is likely to die within the next 6 months if the terminal illness follows its anticipated course, finalizes the prognosis, and is a difficult shift for physicians.[25] Until the patient or family raises the question of medical futility, studies show extensive medical technology will be utilized by physicians to maintain a patient's hope, as is illustrated in ICU admissions.[26]

At the same time, researchers found most patients and caregivers preferred honest and accurate information, provided with empathy and understanding.[27,28] Despite these findings, physicians are reluctant to refer and as the gatekeeper to hospice, create access barriers.[29–31] With many physicians reticent to suggest hospice, sometimes accusing nurses of overstepping their boundaries when responding to family requests for hospice information, ICU nurses are reluctant to engage in what may devolve into a potentially adversarial situation. The result is that patients and their families defer to their physicians' expertise; hospice is suggested in the final days or hours of life.[32–35]

System Barriers

The hospice enrollment decision can be difficult because most insurers (eg, Medicare) require patients to forego life-sustaining treatment to obtain hospice services. Patients are forced to choose between life-sustaining treatments, such as chemotherapy, radiation, blood transfusions, and costly palliative treatments such as intrathecal infusions, and hospice.[36,37] In addition, a system deficit is the entire healthcare team's discomfort with discussing bad news, resulting in avoidance of discussions on EOL care. Moreover, many nurses lack specific training on the delivery of bad news or how to discuss EOL goals in their basic nursing school curriculae.[38] As a result, ICU nurses lack confidence in their communication skills with on-the-job-training their only instruction on delivery of bad news. This lack of proficiency leads the nurse to respond in nontherapuetic ways, such as giving false reassurance "that everything is going to be OK." Unfortunately, all too frequently even during serious healthcare crisis, suboptimal discussions occur, with missed opportunities to conduct in-depth discussions about what the family really wants or to learn their understanding of care preferences.[39] Furthermore, many studies have identified the moral distress in ICU nurses over disagreements about do not resuscitate orders, level of aggressiveness in treatment, and ethical decisions comparing nurses with physicians.[40,41]

NURSES' ROLE

Armed with this knowledge on barriers to hospice and the moral distress caused by lack of congruence with treatment plans for elderly, terminally ill patients admitted to the ICU, the ICU nurse must feel empowered to change the way care is provided to those with life-threatening illness. The nurse must leverage his or her time with the patients' family to facilitate discussions about end-stage disease care (**Table 1**). Inherent in these discussions are finding the words to introduce hospice as an option on the care continuum. The ICU nurse must feel as comfortable in starting these difficult conversations as the daily administration of sophisticated bedside technology. With the relatives of the ICU patient becoming proxy decision makers, the nurse can create an environment that fosters conversation about EOL care planning. With the close, trusting relationship that is prevalent between the nurse and patients' family, the nurse picks up on the subtle cues the families' express and their uncertainty with future treatment plans. The nurse's words matter. For example, when the patient's spouse asks if the patient is going to get better this time, the nurse must see this as an opportunity to start an open dialogue about terminal, incurable illness and what the goals are in continuing treatment.

Surrogate decision makers find their role difficult because they are not familiar with how prognosis is determined in advanced chronic illness states. There are 3 primary trajectories in chronic, irreversible illness; all are based on functional status and time alive.[42] The first trajectory, which is typical in a cancer diagnosis, is a relatively stable period where the patient enjoys minimal decline, followed by a short and rapid decline, often culminating in death in a matter of months once the precipitous decline begins.

The second trajectory is one with intermittent serious, healthcare crises, often marked with hospital admissions and ICU stays, such as with heart and lung failure diseases. Death usually occurs 2 to 5 years after the decline begins, yet, seems "sudden." The third is a prolonged, slow decline with relatively stable health and a lack of acute serious illnesses, as in the second trajectory, yet progressive irreversible deficits in functional capacity such as seen with dementia. This is the patient who gradually loses all independence in activities of daily living, requiring full support. Death in this case is the least predictable, with wide variation from 5 to 8 years after the disease is diagnosed.

Along with disease trajectory, the ICU nurse reviews functional status in preparation for EOL care planning. Also called performance status, this refers to physiologic status, and is defined as one's ability to care for oneself and participate in daily activities. One such scale—the Palliative Performance Scale—is commonly used in hospice and palliative care programs.[43] The scale provides a percentage score from 0% (death) to 100% based on categories of ambulation, activity, evidence of disease impact, self-care ability, and nutritional intake to consciousness level. For example, a score of 10% (common in ICU) is a patient totally bedbound, unable to do any work with extensive evidence of disease, requiring total assistance with hygiene, receiving mouth care only and no oral nutrition or fluids, and is drowsy or comatose.

NURSING INTERVENTIONS

With nursing's holistic approach, the ICU nurse is well-positioned to put together the clinical story of the patient's disease trajectory, performance status, prognosis, and recovery potential in a way the family can picture the likely outcome. Although the family may not initially see the trajectory that the nurse describes or feel comfortable starting the discussion themselves, it is the proverbial "elephant in the room."

The ICU nurse should view the EOL discussion as a critical element in the care plan for the patient with end-stage disease in the ICU. The nurse can guide the discussion to identify the families' understanding of the disease progression, the patient's current functional status, and the likelihood of returning to prehospitalization status. In this

Table 1
Examples of response to use with families of ICU patients, using "dad" as the patient

Family Cue When More Information is Needed	Suggested Response
Disease trajectory/goals	
My dad seems like he is not getting better this time and he would not like to be like this. What more can be done for him?	Can you tell me what your doctor has been saying about your father's illness?
I don't know how my dad is really doing. Do you think he will go home?	Tell me how things have been going before this hospitalization. What was your dad able to do? Did he need help with dressing, meals or bathing?
	If your dad could talk now, what would he tell us about how he wants to live?
	It sounds like your dad may have discussed with you what he would want if he became very sick, did he ever complete an advance directive—a living will? Did he ever talk to you about his preferences for quality of life?
Disease stage	
My dad has been in and out of the hospital for the last year. He always pulls through, but this time he looks the worse.	Tell me about your dad's previous hospitalizations over the last year.
Do you think he is going to get better this time?	From what you have told me, your dad has been sick for many years. He has had 4 hospitalizations in the last year, and each time has had a harder time recovering. In fact, you mentioned that he can't do things for himself like he used to and is getting more and more dependent on you. He frequently talks about how he valued his independence and didn't like to be a burden. For most patients with advanced chronic disease, the course is one of overall decline. (Describe specific symptoms of end-stage disease for the particular patient, such as age, weight loss, minimal responsiveness, oxygen dependence, inability to do activities of daily living, and feeding tube for nutrition). Your dad is very, very sick.
	Most people do not understand what it means to have "everything done." The possibility of surviving CPR is low. Even when CPR is done in the hospital, it often it results in broken ribs and the need for a ventilator (breathing machine); it is not like on TV. If the person survives, they are usually even sicker and require more treatments and procedures than before the CPR was done to stay alive.

(continued on next page)

Table 1
(continued)

Family Cue When More Information is Needed	Suggested Response
If I don't do everything that can be done, I feel like I am giving up on my dad.	It is important for us to honor your dad's wishes and preferences for care. Sometimes we have to change what we are hoping for, and perhaps you are saying that you are hoping your dad's pain and suffering can be reduced. I think I understand your main goal is for your dad to be comfortable.
Performance status	
My dad is not sick enough for hospice.	Your dad is very sick and is showing significant decline. It is unlikely that he will go back to the same way he was before coming into the hospital. Some families come to the point where they decide they do not want to have any further tests or procedures; rather, they want a comfort care model of care. Other families want everything possibly done. How do you feel about these 2 options?
	It is not too early to consider hospice for your dad. As difficult as this may be to hear, your dad meets the criteria for hospice care. His illness has progressed to what we categorize as end stage. Although an exact prognosis is impossible to predict, it is likely your dad will continue to decline, and unlikely that he will recover to do what he could do before he came to the hospital. Your dad is eligible to receive the care that hospice specializes in, taking care of patients whose goals are to be comfortable without all kinds of medical procedures, through an expert medical team that focuses on the entire family, not just the patient.
Dad is not ready for hospice, it is too early.	Standard medical care is focused on curing at all costs, even if it means the quality of life will be poor. In fact, some treatments are really not going to help and may make your dad feel worse or quite uncomfortable. Comfort care focuses on helping the patient feel as good as he can. Hospice does not help patients die sooner; rather, hospice helps people die naturally.

Decision process/advanced care planning	
This is too hard for me to decide what to do.	I can't imagine how difficult this is for you. Most families have a hard time making a decision—it can feel like an enormous responsibility. Why don't you think this over?
Does hospice enrollment mean my dad will have to go somewhere?	I will be here to answer your questions when you are ready. Your dad will receive excellent care no matter what you decide.
What can I expect if I decide to enroll my dad in hospice?	Studies have shown that families found the 24-hour support of hospice, available either by telephone or in person, to be very helpful and they wished they had been more aware and understood what hospice offers. Further, choosing hospice does not mean you can't change your mind later. Enrolling now gives you a support system, and the resources that can be put in motion for the help you need before a crisis situation occurs.
	Hospice is not a place. It is a way of delivering healthcare for a patient who has end-stage disease, in whatever setting the patient is at or can be discharged to (home, nursing home, residential hospice center).
	A hospice team member will contact you to arrange for your dad's enrollment into hospice. The hospice team will work with your dad's doctor and the ICU staff to have a plan which manages your dad's symptoms while honoring his wishes and a comfort care model.

Abbreviations: CPR, cardiopulmonary resuscitation; ICU, intensive care unit.

discussion, the nurse asks questions that create the big picture of what the patient was able to do immediately before hospitalization (level of independence with activities of daily living such as dressing, feeding, toileting, and transfers), their knowledge of disease stage (how long has patient been sick, what they know about the patient's current medical condition and frequency of exacerbations) against the patient's quality of life preferences (What would the patient tell us if they were able to communicate? Did you ever talk about advanced directives or a living will?). The nurse can also overcome misperceptions about medical treatments and what they can achieve toward the family's overall perception of recovery. For example, in an end-stage dementia patient, the family may be considering parenteral tube feedings and intravenous fluids when the patient has stopped eating and drinking. The patient's disease is the underlying reason for the patient's inability to eat and drink, and this information needs to be communicated in a way the family can make a fully informed decision of what they hope to achieve.

EOL CARE PLANNING

Predicting survival is not precise when discussing advanced illness. However, by obtaining a clear understanding of what the family knows, the episodes of serious illness that have transpired over the last several weeks, months, and years, combined with the functional changes that have taken place, the ICU nurse can feel confident with leading a discussion on EOL care. The nurse can describe the current clinical situation, summarize the typical disease trajectory, and educate the family on the meaning of performance status with respect to recovery and planning for the future. Linking the factors associated with long-term prognosis, the ICU nurse can then ask questions to learn the patients' and families' preferences for quality of life. The ICU nurse uses empathy and compassion in her communication, while gently clarifying what is most important to the family, honoring the patient's preferences for EOL care.[43]

The nurse can acknowledge the downhill course and help the family to describe their goals in the context of chronic, irreversible, advanced disease. The nurse can acknowledge the families emotions, support the values that were most important to the patient, and through effective communication advocate for hospice.[44] Based on the family's readiness, the ICU nurse can shift the discussion from the traditional medical model of exhausting technology and medical advances to gain more time, to one of making the most of the time one has left, a comfort care model. The nurse can deploy communication strategies and advocacy to work with physicians and families uncomfortable with discussions on dying. Having first-hand insight on family dynamics, the ICU nurse can weave the comprehensive scope of the hospice team into the discussion, reaching out to the entire families' needs, not just the patient's.

FUTURE DIRECTIONS

When the nurse listens to what is most important to the patient and family the likelihood of transitioning to hospice is greater. Although arguably one of the most difficult decisions a patient or family has to make, the ICU nurse can be instrumental in influencing the decision to enroll in hospice. Through the use of stellar communication skills, the nurse can overcome the barriers in hospice discussions. Likewise, the nurse can intervene with physicians when a referral is indicated and not forthcoming. Facilitating patient empowerment and advocating for patients are hallmarks of good nursing care: Doing the right thing, at the right time, for the right reason.

Our healthcare system is poised to embark on a radical path of change with the passage of the Patient Protection and Affordable Care Act of 2010, with a clear emphasis on decreasing the fragmentation of care. This legislative-driven imperative to a seamless continuum of care requires patients to receive the most appropriate care at the most appropriate time. Hospice should be an integral component of the continuum. Yet, as this article and others have demonstrated, physicians are the gatekeepers to hospice and, when EOL conversations are delayed until patients ask for advanced medical technology to be discontinued, the result is often a difficult death. The Dartmouth Atlas Project[45] found that many clinical teams aggressively treat patients with curative attempts they may not want, at the expense of worsening the quality of their life in their last weeks and months. Nurses can be instrumental with this issue of how to serve patients sooner in the course of their illness, because we are uniquely positioned to have key conversations with patients, families, and physicians. Through essential strategies of education, advocacy, and communication, nurses can impact the hospice decision before the brink of death.

SUMMARY

A key factor in nurses' experiencing moral distress is their feeling of powerlessness to initiate discussions about code status, EOL issues, or patients' preferences.[46] Moreover, nurses encounter physicians who give patients and their families a false picture of recovery or, worse, block EOL discussions from occurring. Since its release in 1995, the landmark study of almost 10,000 patients in the Study to Understand Prognoses and Preferences for Outcomes and Risks of Treatments (SUPPORT) reported a widespread gap with physicians' discussions in honest prognosis and EOL issues. Since the SUPPORT report, other studies have validated patients' and their families' preference for realistic discussions of disease trajectory and life expectancy.[47] Unfortunately, the phenomenon of physicians failing to discuss bad news or terminal disease trajectory persists. Moreover, with a burgeoning geriatric population, coupled with advances in medical treatments, a growing segment of chronically ill patients are admitted to the ICU.

With these communication shortcomings, it becomes an essential element of practice for the ICU nurse to initiate discussions about healthcare goals, preferences, and choices. The ICU nurse must be integral in fostering those discussions, particularly in cases where the family asks if hospice should be considered. Nurses have a long history of patient advocacy, with both the American Nurses Association and the American Association of Critical-Care Nurses stating that nurses have a duty to educate and promote dialogue about patients' preferences, goals, and EOL issues.[48,49] With these tenets in the forefront, the ICU nurse is an integral member of the healthcare team, working with patients and their families to distinguish between what can be done and what should be done.

Too often, hospice is thought of as a last resort. Rather, it is a model of care that centers on the belief that each of us has the right to die pain free and with dignity, and that our families will receive the necessary support to allow us to do so. Despite the high satisfaction reported by decedents of hospice enrollees, 35% of all hospice patients die within 7 days of enrollment owing to late referrals. An ICU stay presents the perfect opportunity to weave EOL care planning into the fabric of everyday patient care. Clearly, the ICU setting cares for the very sickest patients, and knowing what patients and families desire must take precedence in all treatment decisions. The ICU nurse should be proficient in communication skills, using evidence-based communication related to functional status, performance scales, disease trajectory, and prognosis. ICU nurses recognize that not every patient survives their ICU stay; yet, for those patients who will not survive, every ICU nurse wants their patient to experience a "good death." Hospice and the palliative care are important aspects of our care continuum and should not be ignored until the last days or hours of a patient's life. Recognizing eligibility for hospice and its alignment with patient EOL preferences can result in optimal EOL care.

REFERENCES

1. National Hospice and Palliative Care Organization (NHPCO). 2010 NHPCO Facts and figures: hospice care in America. Available at: http://www.nhpco.org/files/public/Statistics_Research/Hospice_Facts_Figures_Oct-2010.pdf. Accessed October 7, 2011.
2. Angus DC, Barnato AE, Linde-Zwirble WT, et al. Use of intensive care at the end of life in the United States: an epidemiologic study. Crit Care Med 2004;32:638–43.
3. Elpern EH, Covert B, Kleinpell R. Moral distress of staff nurses in a medical intensive care unit. Am J Crit Care 2005;14:523–30.
4. Field MJ, Cassell CK, eds. Institute of Medicine Report: approaching death: improving care at the end of Life. Washington, DC: National Academy Press; 1997:4.
5. Rickerson E, Harrold J, Kapo J, et al. Timing of hospice referral and families' perceptions of services: Are earlier hospice referrals better? Am Geriatr Soc 2005;53:819–23.
6. Cherlin E, Fried T, Prigerson H, et al. Communication between physicians and family caregivers about care at the end of life: when do discussions occur and what is said? J Palliat Med 2005;8:1176–85.
7. Finestone A, Inderwies G. Death and dying in the US: barriers to the benefits of palliative and hospice care. Clin Interventions Aging 2008;3:595–9.
8. Boucher J, Bova C, Sullivan-Bolyai T, et al. Next of kin's perspectives of end-of-life care. J Hospice Palliat Nurs 2010;12:41–50.
9. Chapin R, Gordon T, Landry S, et al. Hospice use by older adults knocking on the door of the nursing facility: implications for social work practice. J Soc Work End Life Palliat Care 2007;3:19–37.
10. Feeg VD, Elebiary H. Exploratory study on end-of-life issues: barriers to palliative care and advanced directives. Am J Hospice Palliat Care 2005;22:119–24.
11. Quill T, Norton S, Shah M, et al. What is most important for you to achieve?: an analysis of patient responses when receiving palliative care consultation. J Palliat Med 2006;9:382–8.
12. Casarett DJ, Crowley RL, Stevenson C, et al. Making difficult decisions about hospice enrollment: what do patients and families want to know? J Am Geriatr Soc 2005;53:249–54.
13. Russell K, LeGrand S. "I'm not that sick!" Overcoming the barriers to hospice discussions. Cleve Clin J Med 2006;73:517–24.
14. Lorenz K, Asch S, Rosenfeld K, et al. Hospice admission practices: where does hospice fit in the continuum of care? J Am Geriatr Soc 2004;52:725–30.
15. Lorenz K, Lynn J, Dy S, et al. Evidence for improving palliative care at the end of life: a systematic review. Ann Internal Med 2008;148:147–59.
16. Lynn J. Serving patients who may die soon and their families: the role for hospice and other services. JAMA 2001;285:925–32.
17. Casarett D, Quill TE. "I'm not ready for hospice": strategies for timely and effective hospice discussions. Ann Intern Med 2007;146:443–9.
18. Welch L, Miller S, Martin E, et al. Referral and timing of referral to hospice care in nursing homes: the significant role of staff. Gerontologist 2008;48:477–84.

19. Rhodes R, Mitchell S, Miller S, et al. Bereaved family members' evaluation of hospice care: what factors influence overall satisfaction with services? J Pain Symptom Manage 2008;35:365–71.
20. Casarett D, Crowley R, Hirschman K. How should clinicians describe hospice to patients and families? J Am Geriatr Soc 2004;52:1923–8.
21. Hancock K, Clayton JM, Parker SM, et al. Truth-telling in discussion prognosis in advanced life-limiting illnesses: a systematic review. Palliat Med 2007;21:507–17.
22. McGorty EK, Bornstein BH. Barriers to physicians' decisions to discuss hospice: insights gained from the United States hospice model. J Eval Clin Pract 2003;9: 363–72.
23. Huskamp H, Keating N, Malin J, et al. Discussions with physicians about hospice among patients with metastatic lung cancer. Arch Intern Med 2009;169:954–62.
24. Glare PA, Sinclair CT. Palliative medicine review: prognostication. J Palliat Med 2008;11:84–103.
25. Christakis NA, Iwashyna TJ. Impact of individual and market factors on the timing of initiation of hospice terminal care. Med Care 2000;38:528–41.
26. Gawande A. Letting go. The New Yorker. August 2, 2010. Available at: http://www.newyorker.com/reporting/2010/08/02/100802fa. Accessed October 22, 2011.
27. Andershed B. Relatives in end-of-life care-part 1: a systematic review of the literature for the last five years, January 1999-February 2004. J Clin Nurs 2006;15:1158–70.
28. Innes S, Payne S. Advanced cancer patients' prognostic information preferences: a review. Palliat Med 2009;23:29–39.
29. Brickner L, Scannell K, Marquet S, et al. Barriers to hospice care and referrals: survey of physicians' knowledge, attitudes and perceptions in a health maintenance organization. J Palliat Med 2004;7:411–8.
30. Ogle K, Mavis B, Wang T. Hospice and primary care physicians: attitudes, knowledge, and barriers. Am J Hospice Palliat Care 2003;20:41–51.
31. Kelly K, Thompson M, Waters R. Improving the way we die: a coorientation study assessing agreement/disagreement in the organization -public relationship of hospices and physicians. J Health Commun 2006;11, 607–27.
32. Teno JM, Shu JE, Casarett D, et al. Timing of referral to hospice and quality of care: length of stay and bereaved family members' perceptions of the timing of hospice referral. J Pain Symptom Manage 2007;34:120–5.
33. Rickerson E, Harrold J, Kapo J, et al. Timing of hospice referral and families' perceptions of services: are earlier hospice referrals better? Am Geriatr Soc 2005;53: 819–23.
34. Rhodes R, Mitchell S, Miller S, et al. Bereaved family members' evaluation of hospice care: what factors influence overall satisfaction with services? J Pain Symptom Manage 2008;35:365–71.
35. Jennings B, Ryndes T, D'Onofrio C, et al. Hastings Center Report Special Supplement access to hospice care: expanding boundaries, overcoming barriers 2003;33:s3–59.
36. Vig E, Starks H, Taylor J, et al. Why don't patients enroll in hospice? Can we do anything about it? J Gen Intern Med 2010;25:1009–19.
37. Casarett D, Van Ness PH, O'Leary JR, et al. Are patient preferences for life-sustaining treatment really a barrier to hospice enrollment for older adults with serious illness? J Am Geriatr Soc 2006;54:472–8.
38. Paice JA, Ferrell BR, Coyle N, et al. Global efforts to improve palliative care: the international end-of-life nursing education consortium training programme. J Adv Nurs 2008;61:173–80.

39. Schulman-Green D, McCorkle R, Cherlin E, et al. Nurses' communication of progno-sis and implications for hospice referral: a study of nurses caring for terminally ill hospitalized patients. Am J Crit Care 2005;14:64–70.
40. Cherlin E, Fried T, Prigerson H, et al. Communication between physicians and family caregivers about care at the end of life: when do discussions occur and what is said? J Palliat Med 2005;8:1176–85.
41. Kirchhoff, K. Promoting a peaceful death in the ICU. Crit Care Nurs Clin North Am 2002;14:201–6.
42. Murray SA, Kendall M, Boyd K, Sheikh A. Illness trajectories and palliative care. BMJ 2008;330:218–27.
43. Wilner LS, Arnold RW. The Palliative Performance Scale #125. J Palliat Med 2006;9: 994.
44. Reinke LF, Shannon SE, Engelberg R, et al. Nurses' identification of important yet under-utilized end-of-life care skills for patients with life-limiting or terminal illness. J Palliat Med 2010;13:753–9.
45. Dartmouth Atlas Project (2010). Quality of end-of-life cancer care for Medicare beneficiaries. Available at: http://www.dartmouthatlas.org/downloads/reports/Cancer_report_11_6_10.pdf. Accessed October 25, 2011.
46. Wittenberg-Lyles E, Goldsmith J, Ragan S. The COMFORT initiative: palliative nursing and the centrality of communication. J Hospice Palliat Nurs 2010;12:282–91.
47. Zuzelo PR. Exploring the moral distress of registered nurses. Nurs Ethics 2007;14: 345–59.
48. The SUPPORT principal Investigators. A controlled trial to improve care for seriously ill hospitalized patients: the Study to Understand Prognoses and Preferences for Outcomes and Risks of Treatments (SUPPORT). JAMA 1995;274:1591–8.
49. American Association of Critical-Care Nurses. Scope and standards for acute and critical care nursing practice. Available at: http://www.aacn.org/WD/Practice/Docs/130300-Standards_for_Acute_and_Critical_Care_Nursing.pdf. Accessed October 20, 2011.

Understanding the Neurobiology, Assessment, and Treatment of Substances of Abuse and Dependence: A Guide for the Critical Care Nurse

Vanessa Genung, PhD, RN, PMH-NP-BC, LCSW-ACP, LMFT, LCDC

KEYWORDS

- Neurobiology • Substance abuse • Substance dependence
- Critical care • Acute care • Mesolimbic dopamine system
- Neurochemical dysregulation • Pleasure/reward pathway

Nurses in all arenas of health care encounter and treat patients with alcohol and substance abuse issues. Nurses are in a unique position as front line health care workers to recognize substance abuse problems and educate, treat, and refer.[1] Drug use and abuse can cause serious medical complications that often lead to emergency room treatment, and in many cases, admission to hospitals and critical care units. In 1992 the US Department of Health and Human Services initiated a system of monitoring drug-related emergency room visits through the Office of Applied Studies of the Substance Abuse and Mental Health Services Administration's (SAMHSA) Drug Abuse Warning Network (DAWN).[2] The DAWN report tallies incidences of drug- and alcohol-related accidents, traumas, overdose, detoxification, and withdrawal.[3]

More than a quarter of Americans aged 18 years or older have a diagnosable mental disorder in a given year.[4] And, a silent epidemic contributing to increasing health problems is to be found in the rising numbers of elderly in that nearly 15% of persons over 60 are admitted to acute hospital care affected by alcohol.[5–7] Nearly half of the US adult population will experience some mental disorder in their lifetime.[8] The World Health Organization (WHO) has reported 2008 estimates reflecting that at least 15.3 million persons have drug use disorders, harmful use of alcohol results in 2.5 million deaths each year, 320.000 15- to 29-year-olds die from alcohol-related

The author has nothing to disclose.
Wilson School of Nursing, Midwestern State University, 3410 West Taft Boulevard, Bridwell Hall, Wichita Falls, TX 76308, USA
E-mail address: vanessa.genung@mwsu.edu

Crit Care Nurs Clin N Am 24 (2012) 117–130
doi:10.1016/j.ccell.2012.01.007
0899-5885/12/$ – see front matter © 2012 Elsevier Inc. All rights reserved.

causes—9% of all deaths in that age group, 155 to 250 million of the world's population aged 15 to 64 use psychoactive substances, and injecting drug use is reported in 148 countries, of which 120 report human immunodeficiency virus (HIV) infection among the population.[9] The scope and seriousness of the morbidity and mortality of alcohol and drug use by youth cannot be overestimated or overemphasized.[10,11] This article reviews the neurobiology of addiction and identifies the continuum of nursing care possible in the critical care setting.

THE PATHOLOGIC CYCLE OF ADDICTION

Why would someone abuse a drug? Chemical dependency, although moralized, is a disease of the brain. For many persons it is a result of genetic vulnerability. For others it is influenced by drug use or an outcome of environmental influences. The term *vulnerability* refers to the pathologic condition of neurotransmitters and brain circuit system susceptibility to the influence of a particular drug action. In some cases this vulnerability leads to a predisposition for drug dependency. The formula for drug use/abuse becomes this: environmental influence/genetic vulnerability + drug use = dysregulation of the neurotransmitter system. Dysregulation occurs under continued exposure of the particular brain circuit neurotransmitter system to the drug of choice (DOC). This repeated exposure of the brain circuit nervous system to the DOC leads to adaptive changes in nerve functions referred to as neuroadaptations. Neuroadaptations occurring at the nerve cell receptor site as a result of drug exposure reach a threshold of intolerability leading to an aggressive or compulsive requirement for the drug. Repeated uses of the DOC when it is an illegal substance or when it causes physical, social, or psychological impairment is termed *drug abuse*. Repeated use of a drug of abuse leads to dependency. The individual begins to experience impairment of control to stop using or seeking the DOC and becomes dependent on the drug to produce a certain pathophysiologic relief or experience. When individuals abstain from the DOC, they may experience strong physical or psychological urges to access the drug. These urges are the dependency aspect of addiction. The formula for addiction becomes this: drug use + neuroadaptation = dysregulation + chronic relapse and return. Multiple dysregulations then can lead to polysubstance abuse and dependence.

People have DOCs because when they use, the drugs connect to specific dysregulated neurotransmitter brain circuit systems. The four major classes of abused drugs: stimulants (cocaine, amphetamines, methamphetamines), opiates (heroin, morphine, opium), ethanol, and nicotine cause increased dopamine (DA) transmission in the limbic system—each by different mechanisms. Other commonly abused drugs include cannabinoids (marijuana, hashish), club drugs (ecstasy [3,4-methylenedioxymethamphetamine; MDMA], flunitrazepam [Rohypnol], gamma-hydroxybutyric acid [GHB]), dissociative drugs (ketamine, phencyclidine [PCP], salvia, dextromethorphan), hallucinogens (lysergic acid diethylamide [LSD], mescaline, psilocybin), other compounds (steroids, inhalants), and prescription drugs (central nervous system depressants, benzodiazepines, stimulants, and opioids).[12–15]

NEUROBIOLOGY OF ADDICTION

What are the major neurotransmitters involved in drugs of abuse? The two primary portions of the brain involved in addictions are the neocortex and the limbic system. Neocortex development helps us differentiate between reality and fantasy and is therefore a primary sorter of rational thought and discrimination between ordinary experience and risk-taking and the neocortex is often involved in romantic, sexual, or mystical thought or exaggerations of these in the form of psychosis. The neurotransmitters that are known to be involved in this area of the brain include: DA, serotonin (5HT), norepinephrine (NE), and phenylethylamine.[12–14] Drugs of abuse mimic or imitate the brain's neurotransmitters and increase neurotransmitters that regulate pleasure. Drugs of abuse that are known to influence the neocortex include LSD, tetrahydrocannabinol (THC), and cannabis.[16,17] The limbic system of the brain integrates thought and emotion and is responsible for senses of arousal and satiation.[16] When DA and adrenalin charge the limbic structures, the person experiences arousal. In excess, the person experiences euphoria or mania and often loses some level of rational capacity. This loss of capacity may lead to addictive or risk-taking behaviors. Drugs that are known to influence this area include cocaine, amphetamines, diet pills, and MDMA (ecstasy).[12–14,16] At the other end of the spectrum, when gamma aminobutyric acid (GABA) and endorphins are activated in this area the mind quiets, and to excess the person experiences apathy, anhedonia, avolition, and depression. To that end the individual may seek remedies such as food, alcohol, drugs, sedatives, pain pills, or opiates to feel better or feel good again.[16] **Fig. 1** displays the brain circuitry involved in pathways of drug reward and addiction.

NEUROTRANSMITTER DRUG AND MENTAL HEALTH EFFECTS

What drugs affect which neurotransmitters? There are many neurotransmitters in the brain; however, the most pertinent to drug addiction are those that innervate the

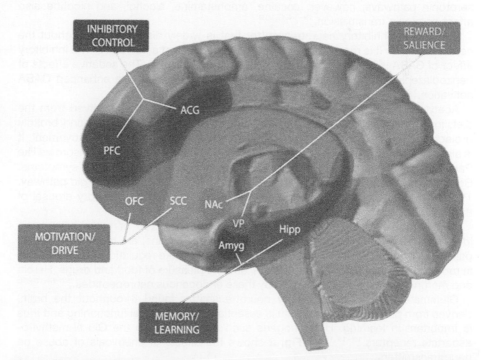

Fig. 1. Circuits involved in drug abuse and addiction. All of these brain regions must be considered in developing strategies to effectively treat addiction. ACG, anterior cingulate gyrus; Amyg, amygdala; Hipp, hippocampus; NAc, nucleus accumbens; OFC, orbitofrontal cortex; PFC, prefrontal cortex; SCC, subcallosal cingulate; VP, ventral posterior. (*Courtesy of* the National Institute on Drug Abuse, Bethesda, MD.)

neocortex and the limbic system, the reward pathway. Because addiction often occurs in combinations of substances of abuse and with other mental health issues, the interconnectedness and broad impact of neuronal dysfunction are an issue.

DA is derived from tyrosine and is structurally related to NE. It is involved in movement, learning, pleasure, and motivation. There are five DA pathways: meso-cortical (cortex), mesolimbic (limbic), nigrostriatal (basal ganglia), tuberoinfundibular (pituitary), and the mysterious fifth (thalamus). The mesolimbic dopamine pathway projects from the ventral tegmental area (VTA) to the nucleus accumbens. This path is considered the reward path and is activated by most substances of abuse. It is also the path most likely to be activated in mental health issues such as mania and psychosis.[12–14,16–19]

NE is also derived from tyrosine and is found in the locus coeruleus, from there projecting broadly throughout the brain. It is responsible for arousal and response to stress. Cocaine and amphetamines affect the transmission of NE and contribute to the stimulating and pleasurable effects of these drugs. It is also the path most likely activated in mental health issues such as attention-deficit/hyperactivity disorder and anxieties.[12–14,16–19]

Derived from tryptophan, 5HT initiates in the midbrain raphe nuclei and broadly projects throughout the cortex, hypothalamus, and limbic system. Additional 5HT receptors are to be found in the gut, platelets, and spinal cord. It is also the path most likely to be involved in pain, movement, sleep, appetite, anxiety, and depressive mood mental health disturbances. LSD and ecstasy have their primary effects in the serotonin pathways; however, cocaine, amphetamine, alcohol, and nicotine also affect serotonin transmission.[12–14,16–19]

GABA is an inhibitory neurotransmitter that is widely distributed throughout the nervous system. It is responsible for slowing the activity of a nerve cell. The inhibitory effect of GABA is involved in anxiety, agitation, and seizures. The sedative effects of benzodiazepines, barbiturates, and alcohol are accomplished via enhanced GABA activation.[12–14,16–19]

Acetylcholine (ACh) is a neurotransmitter formed from choline, derived from the diet, involving coenzyme A. ACh initiates in the basal ganglia nucleus and broadly projects throughout the cortex. It plays a role in learning, memory, and movement. It is also the DA path most likely to be involved in mental health movement disorders like Parkinson disease, memory disorders like dementia, and extrapyramidal symptoms. Both nicotinic and muscarinic receptors are to be found in the cholinergic pathway. Thus, ACh is implicated in nicotine dependence and has a contributory arousal of thought with the use of cocaine and amphetamine.[12–14,16–18]

Neuropeptides connect chains of amino acids, and 200 or more have been identified in the brain. Opioid peptides, primarily endorphins, are the body's natural pain killers. Neuropeptides manage food and water intake regulation and play a role in modulating anxiety, pain, reproduction, and the pleasure of food and drugs. Heroin and morphine bind to receptors used by these endogenous neuropeptides.[12–14,16–18]

Glutamate (Glu) is an excitatory neurotransmitter found throughout the brain, derived from proteins in the diet. Glu is essential in hippocampal functioning and thus is important in learning. Hallucinogens such as PCP act on the Glu N-methyl-D-aspartate receptors.[12–14,16–19] **Fig. 2** shows the effects of chemicals of abuse on neurotransmitters.

RAPID ASSESSMENT

How do I tell if someone has an alcohol or drug problem? To identify drug use early in medical settings, the National Institute on Drug Abuse (NIDA) recommends

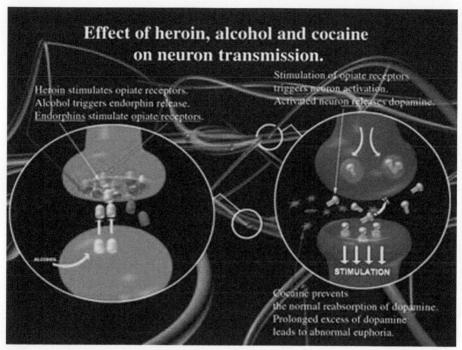

Fig. 2. The effects of heroin, alcohol, and cocaine on neuron transmission. (*Courtesy of* the National Institute on Drug Abuse, Bethesda, MD.)

screening in a three-step process using the Five A's: Ask, Advise, Assess, Assist, Arrange.[20] Step 1: Ask patients about past drug use of tobacco products, alcohol in many types of beverages, cannabis, cocaine, prescription stimulants, methamphetamine, inhalants, sedatives or sleeping aids, hallucinogens, street opioids, prescription pain meds, and stimulant drinks (coffee, Big Red, Monster energy drinks, Dr Pepper). Step 2: Determine their risk level by assessing their frequency of exposure to substance. Step 3–5: Depending on risk level, provide advice, assess their readiness to change, assist them by offering help, and arrange the assistance by referring them for evaluation and treatment by specialists.[20] **Box 1** presents two traditional rapid assessment tools based on the acronyms CAGE and TWEAK.

SIGNS AND SYMPTOMS OF INTOXIFICATION AND WITHDRAWAL

What will it look like when the patient is intoxicated or withdrawing from a substance? First consider the drug's neurologic classification as an exciter or inhibitor. The brain works like a car, with a gas pedal and a brake pedal to start (excite) and stop (inhibit) neural electric activity. When a drug of abuse is introduced it alters how the brain's motor responds to traffic signals like green-gas-go and red-brake-stop. When a depressant is introduced, the brain engages the brake pedal by enhancing the naturally inhibiting GABA complex and reducing the naturally excitatory activity of Glu. The drug's reinforcing effects occur because of its activity in the brain's mesolimbic DA (MDA) reward pathway. The depressant has additional actions on the brain's opiate and cannabinoid receptors.[12–14] When more of a depressant is introduced, the brain begins the process of slowing down to shutting down, center by

---

Box 1
Rapid screening tests

CAGE

C-Has anyone ever felt you should C-ut down on your drinking?

A-Have people A-nnoyed you by criticizing your drinking?

G-Have you ever felt G-uilty about your drinking?

E-Have you ever had a drink first thing in the morning (E-opener) to steady your nerves or to get rid of a hangover?

+1 = alcohol problem indication, 2+ = alcohol problem

TWEAK

T-olerance (2 pts): How many drinks can you hold? (6+=tolerance)

W-orried (2 pts): Have close friends or relatives worried or complained about your drinking in the past year?

E-ye opener (1 pt): Do you sometimes take a drink in the morning when you first get up?

A-mnesia (1 pt): Has a friend or family member ever told you about things you said or did while you were drinking that you could not remember?

K-cut down (1 pt): Do you sometimes feel the need to cut down on your drinking?

---

center from front to back (thinking to doing) and outside to inside (rational thought to primitive emotional process). The person experiences disinhibition of judgment, reduced censorship of verbalizations, and ultimately sedation. This scenario is intoxication on a depressant: extreme neurologic inhibition. Depressant intoxication to extremes can cause the brain to shut off and may cause death. When intoxication occurs on a regular basis the brain becomes accustomed to the disinhibiting activity of GABA, the deceleration process. If for some reason the person stops this deceleration suddenly, the brain no longer has the brake on (the depressant substance enhancing GABA) and the brain begins to act as if the gas pedal (Glu) is being pressed and moves into acceleration. GABA is no longer activated to slow brain process down. This scenario is the process of withdrawal from a depressant. See **Table 1** for a list of signs and symptoms of intoxication and withdrawal from a depressant.

Following the same gas-brake analogy, when a stimulant is introduced, the brain engages the gas pedal. When more of a stimulant is introduced, the brain begins the process of speeding up. Stimulants block presynaptic vesicular monoamine transporter (VMAT), noradrenaline active reuptake transporter (NET), and dopamine active reuptake transporter (DAT) thereby increasing the availability of NE and DA to activate postsynaptic nerve conduction.[12–14] When more of a stimulant is introduced, the brain begins the process of speeding up activity from thought to emotions to behavioral activity. The person experiences hyperalertness, expanded thought, increased energy, and pleasure. This scenario is intoxication on a stimulant. Stimulant intoxication to extremes can cause symptoms of mania or psychosis because of the activation of the DA paths in the brain. The accompanying physical excitability is a result of the activation of the NE paths. When the person comes off the stimulant the brain enters rapid deceleration as the amount of NE and DA available for nerve activation drops, producing what might resemble the brake pedal effect. This

Table 1 Clinical presentation and management of depressant drugs of abuse	
Intoxication	**Withdrawal**
☐ Semiconscious	☐ Seizures, death
☐ Slurred speech	☐ Delirium, hallucination
☐ Memory loss	☐ Anxiety, irritability
☐ Flaccid appearance	☐ Generalized tremors
☐ Loss of coordination	☐ Muscle pain
☐ Constricted pupils, glazed eyes	☐ Increased vital signs
☐ Decreased vital signs	☐ Nausea
☐ Nausea, vomiting	☐ Sweating

Management:
Benzodiazepines-chlordiazepoxide (Librium), diazepam (Valium), lorazepam (Ativan) for alcohol withdrawal; naloxone, naltrexone (mu opiate antagonists) to block opiate and alcohol reward; acamprosate (Glu antagonist/GABA agonist) for alcohol deterrent; disulfiram (irreversible aldehyde dehydrogenase antagonist) for alcohol aversion; flumazenil (Romazicon-benzodiazepine antagonist) for benzo reversal, Clonidine (central alpha-2 agonist) to stabilize central nervous system.
Abusive DOC:
Alcohol, opioids, morphine, heroin, benzodiazepines, marijuana.

scenario is the process of withdrawal from a stimulant: rapid deceleration. **Table 2** gives a list of signs and symptoms of intoxication and withdrawal from a stimulant.

Understanding euphorics or hallucinogens requires a different analogy, one viewed through kaleidoscopic glasses. Some euphoric drugs affect the serotonin (primarily 5HT2A) neurotransmitter process, whereas others affect the NE and DA neurotransmitters. What these substances have in common is the associated changes in sensory perception including visual illusions, hallucinations, and an acute awareness of all things great and wonderful. Colors are heard, sounds seen, dreams are real, and time slows. The greater the intoxication the more likely the "bad trip," wherein delirium and disorientation increases; agitation, panic, and fear set in; and ultimately there is the possibility of an acute psychotic break from reality. Because euphoric hallucinogens work on all three major neurotransmitter pathways, predominantly the 5HT

Table 2 Clinical presentation and management of stimulant drugs of abuse	
Intoxication	**Withdrawal**
☐ Anxiety, paranoia, psychosis	☐ Extreme depression, suicide
☐ Rapid speech and thought process	☐ Craving
☐ Insomnia	☐ Anxiety, suspicious
☐ Dilated pupils	☐ Generalized malaise
☐ Increased vital signs	☐ Irritability, agitation, restlessness
☐ Lip smacking	☐ Lack of pleasure
☐ Dry nares, nosebleeds	☐ Vivid/unpleasant dreams
☐ Anorexia	

Management: Benzodiazepines, diazepam, antipsychotics.
Abusive DOC: Cocaine, ice, methylphenidate, amphetamines, methamphetamines.

Table 3	
Clinical presentation and management of euphoric drugs of abuse	
Intoxication	Withdrawal
☐ Anxiety, depression	☐ Craving
☐ Paranoia, ideas of reference	☐ Flu-like symptoms
☐ Hallucinations, illusions	No physical signs except with PCP (violence, muscle rigidity, convulsions, coma)
☐ Synesthesia, depersonalization	
☐ Amnesia	
☐ Poor coordination	
☐ Dilated pupils, blurred vision	
☐ Increased vital signs	
☐ Nausea, vomiting	

Management: Benzodiazepines, charcoal (PCP), beta-blockers.
Abusive DOC: Ecstasy, GHB, LSD, PCP.

paths, and in the reward circuits of VTA and nucleus accumbens they are capable of producing incredible tolerance, even from a single dose.[12–14] And, when the kaleidoscope glasses come off and the drug is gone from the system, the brain may continue to remember the event and in a spontaneous replay, referred to as a flashback, reenact elements of the hallucinated experience. It is hypothesized that the amygdala may play a role in emotionally remembering some elements of the intoxication experience and replay the event. There is no withdrawal from hallucinogens per se, but the possibility of unannounced flashbacks may be the cause of great concern to the user.[12–14] **Table 3** lists signs and symptoms of intoxication and withdrawal from a euphoric.

COMORBIDITY

When there is an overlap of factors such as genetic vulnerability, environmental stress, trauma, drug use, and neurodysregulation, there is fertile ground for comorbidity of mental illness and drug addiction or polysubstance coaddiction. Research has demonstrated a high prevalence of drug use and dependence among individuals with mood and anxiety disorders; a higher prevalence of smoking among patients with any mental disorder, most prominently bipolar disorder and schizophrenia; a higher prevalence of mental disorders among patients with drug use disorders; and a higher risk of adult psychosis in persons who had a genetic vulnerability (COMP val-val) and used cannabis as adolescents.[21, 22] **Table 4** provides a list of coaddiction combinations in neurotransmitters involved in addiction and reward. Note that ethyl alcohol has an effect at every neurotransmitter, the implication being that early drinking can precipitate other substance use or demonstrate a neurotransmitter vulnerability or irregularity.

RISK MANAGEMENT

Who is most vulnerable to substance abuse? Identifying vulnerable persons and recognizing what signs and symptoms to look for are the first steps to prevention and early treatment. Children and adolescents are at risk for mortal or lifelong complications when introduced to drugs of abuse because their neurologic systems are still in development. NIDA has identified the risk factors for youth to be early aggressive

Table 4	
Frequent coaddiction combinations with dysfunctioning neurotransmitter	
DOC-Polysubstance	**Neurotransmitter**
Cocaine	DA
Amphetamines	Dopamine
ETOH	
Opioids	END
ETOH	Endorphins
Nicotine	ACH
ETOH	Acetylcholine
BZD	GABA
ETOH	Gamma-aminobutyric acid
LSD	5HT
ETOH	Serotonin
ETOH	GLU
	Glutamate
ETOH	Substance P
	NK1R
Cannabis	ENCB
ETOH	Endocannabinoids

Abbreviations: BZD, benzodiazepines; ETOH, ethanol (alcohol).

behavior, lack of parental supervision, poverty, drug availability, and substance use. Likewise, NIDA suggests protective factors for youths to include self-control, parental monitoring, strong neighborhood attachment, antidrug use policies, and academic competence.[15] Other populations at risk include the elderly, those dependent on prescription drugs, persons with unmanaged pain, those living in impoverished environments or experiencing traumatic life events, and persons with a genetic predisposition as observed by family members who abuse substances or have mental illness.

TREATMENT AND CARE MANAGEMENT

To whom do you refer a patient for treatment? When substance abuse has been identified in a patient, the person and their family members as a whole are recognized as being in need of treatment. Early recognition and referral are the first steps. Referrals for evaluation can be made to a psychiatric mental health nurse practitioner (PMH-NP), clinical nurse specialist (CNS), advanced practice registered nurse, psychiatrist (medical doctor, MD, or doctor of osteopathy, DO), psychologist, clinical social worker (LCSW-ACP), or licensed professional counselor (LPC). All of these professionals would be masters or doctoral prepared and licensed for working with persons and families with substance abuse issues. Licensed chemical dependency counselors are also trained specialists who work with substance abuse populations. This licensure does not require graduate school preparation.

BEHAVIORAL MANAGEMENT

What type of treatment is available? Specialty evaluation can direct the patient and the family to inpatient or outpatient admission in a drug rehabilitation treatment facility, a detoxification program, cognitive behavior therapy (CBT) program, self-help support groups, and further evaluation. Detoxification programs can be either inpatient or outpatient. Outpatient behavioral programs can be partial hospitalization or day programs and provide counseling, group therapies, 12-step Alcoholics Anonymous/Narcotics Anonymous principles for recovery, CBT, motivational enhancement, interviewing, and contingency management programs. Residential rehabilitation is an intensive live-in recovery program. Other programs include peer to peer coaching and community reinforcement. Medical management refers to the provision of some CBT with pharmacotherapy.[10,14,21]

The NIDA Research Report indicates promising response to behavioral therapies for patients with comorbid conditions.[10,21] Three behavioral treatments are recommended for adolescents: multisystem therapy (MST), brief strategic family therapy (BSFT), and CBT. MST targets peer culture and antisocial attitude. BSFT focuses on conduct issues in the home, family, and school environments. CBT directs attention to maladaptive beliefs and behaviors. In adult populations, five therapeutic venues are reported to show promise: therapeutic communities (TCs), assertive community treatment (ACT), dialectical behavioral therapy (DBT), exposure therapy (ET), and integrated group therapy (IGT). TCs focus on resocialization of the individual. ACT approach involves a more assertive, team-managed, individualized plan for the person. DBT redirects responsibility and focuses choice-making on the person and targets reduction in self-harm behaviors. ET involves repeated exposure to some element to desensitize to a feared event and develop adaptive methods of coping. IGT is a new treatment designed to treat for comorbid bipolar disorder and drug addiction.[6,10,21]

CLINICAL PRESENTATION AND SYMPTOMATIC MANAGEMENT

What medications are used to treat the symptoms of the particular drug? Back to our brake and gas pedals analogies. When a patient is intoxicated on a central nervous system depressant, the brain is shutting down, decelerating, and when detoxing (withdrawing), the brain is accelerating. Treatments are targeted toward medical stabilization during detox, preventing seizure during withdrawals, and reduction of reward or introduction of aversive response upon termination of substance of abuse.

When a patient is intoxicated on a stimulant the brain is in acceleration mode, and when detoxing the brain is decelerating. Treatments are targeted toward medical stabilization, preventing seizures while detoxing, and reducing the acceleration excitement of the DA and NE surge during intoxication.

When a patient is intoxicated on euphoric hallucinogens the brain is in a sensory make-believe Peter Pan land. For many it is a frightening experience of relentless unrealities often revisited in times to come. Treatments are targeted toward medical stabilization, gastrically removing as much of the substance as possible, and psychiatric stabilization by treating for the specific substance introduced. See **Tables 1 to 3** for a review of management strategies for depressant, stimulant, and euphoric substances.

FDA PHARMACOLOGIC-APPROVED TREATMENTS

The US Food and Drug Administration (FDA) has approved three pharmacologic treatments for nicotine, four for alcohol, and four for opioids. Medications that have proved effective work in the affected dysfunctional brain pathways by making drug use aversive, by blocking euphoric effects, or by reducing drug cravings. Kampman[23] itemized the effective medications currently approved by the FDA for treatment of

Table 5 FDA-approved pharmacologic treatments	
Substance	**Treatment**
Nicotine (3)	Nicotine replacement therapy
	Bupropion - Zyban
	Varenicline - Chantix
Alcohol (ETOH) (4)	Disulfiram - Antabuse
	Naltrexone - ReVia
	Acamprosate - Campral
	Depo-Naltrexone - Vivitrol (IM monthly)
Opioids (4)	Methadone
	Buprenorphine - Suboxone, Subutex
	Naltrexone - ReVia

drug and alcohol dependence.[12, 23] For alcohol dependence there are disulfiram, naltrexone (oral and long-acting intramuscular), and acamprosate. For opiate dependence, methadone, buprenorphine, and oral naltrexone are available. For nicotine dependence there are bupropion (Zyban), varenicline (Chantix), and nicotine replacement patches. There are no drugs with current FDA approval for the treatment of stimulant or cannabis dependence.[12, 23] **Table 5** lists the 11 drugs that the FDA has approved for treatment for these substances.

TREATMENT BARRIERS

SAMSHA and NIDA have done several national surveys to identify the state of alcohol and drug abuse treatment initiatives and patient responses. The reasons cited for patients not seeking treatment included cost or insurance barriers, not being ready to stop, wanting to handle it on their own, no transportation, no programming available in the area, they did not want treatment, and they did not know where to go. On the average, not being ready to stop using and cost barriers ranked the highest as barriers to treatment.[24,25]

SUMMARY

What do I as a critical care nurse do? Nurses, by virtue of being trained in health promotion, and also because they interact with patients, families, and communities, have firsthand opportunities to play an active role in practicing primary prevention. To avoid the first occurrence of substance abuse, assess community need, assess facility needs, and identify potential risk. Identify the magnitude of the problem. Intervene early with the youth and at-risk populations. Refer patients and their families to mental health specialists. Provide education to patients, families, communities.[1,26,27] To reduce occurrences of substance abuse, practicing secondary prevention requires prompt action in the earliest moments of recognizing a problem and directing patients to early intervention and rehabilitation. Screening your patients, providing brief education, and prompt referral constitutes early intervention.[1,26,27] To retard the progress of the disease, practice tertiary prevention by providing education, counseling, and support to the afflicted in achieving and maintaining sobriety through medication compliance and rehabilitative group and counseling work.[1,26,27]

The goal of intervention in the lives of substance abusers is to stop drug use, avoid relapse, and sustain recovery. After years of research, NIDA has identified 13 fundamental principles to effective drug abuse treatment.[18]

1. Addiction is a complex but treatable disease that affects brain function and behavior.
2. No single treatment is appropriate for everyone.
3. Treatment needs to be readily available.
4. Effective treatment attends to multiple needs of the individual, not just his or her drug abuse.
5. Remaining in treatment for an adequate period of time is critical.
6. Counseling—individual and/or group—and other behavioral therapies are the most commonly used forms of drug abuse treatment.
7. Medications are an important element of treatment for many patients, especially when combined with counseling and other behavioral therapies.
8. An individual's treatment and services plan must be assessed continually and modified as necessary to ensure it meets his or her changing needs.
9. Many drug-addicted individuals also have other mental disorders that need treatment.
10. Medically assisted detoxification in the first stage of addiction treatment and by itself does little to change long-term drug abuse.
11. Treatment does not need to be voluntary to be effective.
12. Drug use during treatment must be monitored continuously, because lapses during treatment do occur.
13. Treatment programs should assess patients for the presence of HIV/AIDS, hepatitis B and C, tuberculosis, and other infectious diseases, as well as provide targeted risk-reduction counseling to help patients modify or change behaviors that place them at risk of contracting or spreading infectious diseases.

To truly impact this disease, there needs to be improvement in the identification of risk factors and early identification and early intervention with children and adolescents. The future of neuroscience is in objective brain scans and genetic testing. Out of these approaches can come more objective measures of addiction and dependence using brain scans and genetic testing. These measures would potentially allow for the development of vaccines for specific drugs of abuse and dependence, as well as increasingly selective and effective pharmacologic approaches for treatment and a new consensus on standard of care for substance dependence.

RESOURCES

SAMSHA home page: http://www.samhsa.gov/

SAMSHA SBIRT (screening, brief intervention, and referral to treatment) Web site: http://sbirt.samhsa.gov/index.htm

SAMSHA DAWN special topics: http://dawninfo.samhsa.gov/pubs/shortreports/default.asp

SAMHSA's treatment facility locator: http://dasis3samhsa.gov

National Institute of Mental Health (NIMH) home page: http://www.nimh.nih.gov/

NIDA home page: http://www.nida.nih.gov/

NIDA Web sites:

  drugabuse.gov

  backtoschool.drugabuse.gov

  smoking.drugabuse.gov

hiv.drugabuse.gov
marijuana-info.org
clubdrugs.gov
steroidabuse.gov
teens.drugabuse.gov
inhalants.drugabuse.gov
NIDAMED: http://www.drugabuse.gov/NIDAMED
National Institute on Alcohol Abuse and Alcoholism (NIAAA): http://www.niaaa.
   nih.gov
WHO home page: http://www.who.int/en/
WHO The ASSIST Project: http://www.who.int/substance_abuse/activities/assist/
   en/index.html

REFERENCES

1. Nkowane AM, Saxena S. Opportunities for an improved role for nurses in psychoactive substance use: review of the literature. Int J Nurs Pract 2004;10:102–10.
2. Substance Abuse and Mental Health Services Administration, Center for Behavioral Health Statistics and Quality. Drug Abuse Warning Network, 2008: national estimates of drug-related emergency department visits. HHS Publication No. SMA 11–4618. Rockville (MD); 2011.
3. Substance Abuse and Mental Health Administration, Office of Applied Studies. Drug Abuse Warning Network, 2006: national estimates of drug-related emergency department visits. DAWN Series D-30, DHHS Publication No. (SMA) 08–4339. Rockville (MD); 2008.
4. Kessler RC, Chiu WT, Demler O, et al. Prevalence, severity, and comorbidity of 12-month DSM-IV disorders in the National Comorbidity Survey replication. Arch Gen Psychiatry 2005;62:617–27.
5. Kraemer KL, Conigliaro J, Saitz R. Managing alcohol withdrawal in the elderly. Drugs Aging 1999;15(6):409–25.
6. Barrick C, Connors GJ. Relapse prevention and maintaining abstinence in older adults with alcohol-use disorders. Drugs Aging 2002;19(8):583–94.
7. Wallace C, Black JD, Fothergill A. Integrated assessment of older adults who misuse alcohol. Nurs Stand 2010;24(33):51–7.
8. Kessler RC, Berglund P, Demler O, et al. Lifetime prevalence and age-of-onset distributions of DSM-IV disorders in the National Comorbidity Survey Replication. Arch Gen Psychiatry 2005;62:593–602.
9. World Health Organization. Management of substance abuse. Available at: http://www.who.int/substance_abuse/facts/en/. Accessed December 1, 2011.
10. Perepletchikova F, Krystal JH, Kaufman J. Practitioner review: adolescent alcohol use disorders: assessment and treatment issues. J Child Psychol Psychiatry 2008;49(11):1131–54.
11. Elliott ET, Souder CA, Privette T, et al. The scope of adolescent prescription drug abuse. Emergency Medicine 2009;41(1):16–8. Available at: http://www.emedmag.com/html/pre/cov/covers/041010016.asp. Accessed December 1, 2011.
12. Stahl S. Stahl's essential psychopharmacology. 3rd edition. New York: Cambridge University Press; 2008.
13. Schatzberg AF, Nemeroff CB. Textbook of psychopharmacology. 4th edition. Arlington (VA): American Psychiatric Publishing Inc; 2009.
14. Stern TA. Drug addiction. In: Brigido A, Byrne A, editors. Massachusetts general hospital: comprehensive clinical psychiatry. Philadelphia: Mosby Elsevier; 2008. p. 355–69.

15. National Institute on Drug Abuse. Preventing drug abuse among children and adolescents. Available at: http://drugabuse.gov/prevention/risk.html. Accessed December 1, 2011.

16. Milkman HB, Sunderwirth SG. Craving for ecstasy and natural highs: a positive approach to mood alteration. Thousand Oaks (CA): Sage Publications Inc; 2010.

17. National Institute on Drug Abuse. Addiction science: from molecules to managed care. Available at: http://www.nida.nih.gov/pubs/teaching/Teaching6/Teaching1. html. Accessed December 1, 2011.

18. National Institute on Drug Abuse. Drugpages. Available at: http://www.nida.nih.gov/ drugpages/. Accessed December 1, 2011.

19. Stern TA, Rosenbaum JF, Fava M, et al. Alcohol-related disorders. In: Brigido A, Byrne A, editors. Massachusetts general hospital: comprehensive clinical psychiatry. Philadelphia: Mosby Elsevier; 2008. p. 337–54.

20. National Institute on Drug Abuse. Screening for drug use in general medical settings. Quick reference guide. NIH Pub Id: 09-7384. Published April 2009. Available at: http://drugabuse.gov/nidamed/quickref/screening_qr./. Accessed December 1, 2011.

21. National Institute on Drug Abuse. Comorbidity: addiction and other mental illnesses. Research Report Series. NIH Pub Id: 10-5771. Published September 2010. Available at: http://www.nida.nih.gov/researchreports/comorbidity/ or http://www.nationaltasc. org/PDF/RRComorbidity.pdf. Accessed December 1, 2011.

22. Slade M, Taber D, Clark MM, et al. Best practices for the treatment of patients with mental and substance use illnesses in the emergency department. Dis Mon 2007;53: 536–80.

23. Kampman KM. Biologic treatments for drug and alcohol dependence. Prim Psychiatry 2010;17(2):40–5.

24. Substance Abuse and Mental Health Services Administration. The National Survey on Drug Use and Health. Published 2003. Available at: http://www.samhsa.gov/data/ 2k3/SAnoTX/SAnoTX.htm. Accessed December 1, 2011.

25. National Institute on Drug Abuse. NIDA InfoFacts: understanding drug abuse and addiction. Available at: http://wwwl.drugabuse.gov/infofacts/understand.html. Accessed December 1, 2011.

26. Adams KL. Conundrums in the intensive care unit: when substance abuse meets critical illness. AACN News 2005;22(4):12–6.

27. Lopez-Bushnell K, Fassler C. Nursing care of hospitalized medical patients with addictions. J Addict Nurs 2004;15:177–82.

Acute Delirium: Differentiation and Care

Cheryl Holly, EdD, RN[a,b,]*, E. Renee Cantwell, DNP, RN, CNE[b],
Yuri Jadotte, MD[b]

KEYWORDS

- Delirium • Assessment • Prevention • Treatment

Key Points: ACUTE DELIRIUM

- Delirium is a common, preventable condition seen in hospitalized elderly patients.
- Delirium has multiple causes and is usually associated with predisposing factors (visual impairment, alcohol abuse, severe illness) and precipitating factors (immobility, isolation, poor nutrition).
- Health care professionals do not engage in routine assessment of delirium in hospitalized patients.
- Successful management of hospital-acquired delirium is best accomplished using a combination of prevention techniques and early treatment with the onset of symptoms.

OBJECTIVES FOR RECALL

1. Describe the presentation of delirium in hospitalized patients.
2. Distinguish among delirium, depression and dementia.
3. Describe the pathophysiology of intensive care unit delirium as a hospital-acquired condition, including commonly associated risk factors.
4. Describe the steps in assessing for delirium using readily available valid and reliable tools.
5. Describe bundled strategies for prevention and treatment of hospital-acquired delirium.
6. Explain the cognitive, psychological, and quality of life outcomes post intensive care unit delirium.

---

[a] Department of Capacity Building Systems, University of Medicine and Dentistry of New Jersey School of Nursing, 65 Bergen Street, GA 213, Newark, NJ 07101, USA
[b] New Jersey Center for Evidence Based Practice, University of Medicine and Dentistry of New Jersey School of Nursing, 65 Bergen Street, GA 213, Newark, NJ 07101, USA
* Corresponding author. Department of Capacity Building Systems, University of Medicine and Dentistry of New Jersey School of Nursing, 65 Bergen Street, GA 213, Newark, NJ 07101.
E-mail address: hollych@umdnj.edu

Crit Care Nurs Clin N Am 24 (2012) 131–147
doi:10.1016/j.ccell.2012.01.008
0899-5885/12/$ – see front matter © 2012 Elsevier Inc. All rights reserved.

ccnursing.theclinics.com

Delirium, from the ancient Greek *de lira* (off the path), is a disturbance of consciousness characterized by an acute onset, disorganized thinking, and a fluctuating course of inattention.[1] Delirium is also referred to as an acute state of confusion or acute cognitive dysfunction. It is the most common mental health issue found in the general hospital setting, with reports of up to 80% in critical care patients, 60% of whom were either previously comatose and/or were receiving mechanical ventilation.[2] There are further indications that up to half of all admitted older patients experiencing delirium were admitted for treatment of a hip fracture, vascular surgery, or cardiac condition, and that delirium is associated with greater potential for 30- to 90-day readmissions.[3] Adamis and colleagues[4] reported that these rates are likely to be underestimates resulting from bias in recruitment for delirium studies and that actual rates can be much higher. Recently, delirium was reported to be one of the six leading causes of preventable conditions in hospitalized patients older than 65 years.[5]

Delirium has been indicated as a predictor of increased mortality,[6] increased length of stay,[7] increased time on mechanical ventilation,[6] increased hospital costs of up to 40%,[8] increased rates of failed extubation and reintubation,[9,10] increased long-term cognitive impairment leading to dementia in the elderly,[11] and increased instances of discharge to a long-term care facility.[2] Characteristic features include inattention, disorganized thinking, and an altered mental status, sometimes with hallucinations.[12] Delirium is not to be confused with dementia, a state of generalized cognitive deficit in which there is a gradual deterioration of intellectual ability. Dementia usually develops over years and demonstrates levels of cognitive impairment from mild to severe. Nor should delirium be confused with depression, which is also a common misdiagnosis. Depression typically develops over a period of time and is accompanied by feelings of hopelessness and inadequacy to a degree not warranted by circumstances. Depression can lead to an individual's inability to take care of his or her everyday responsibilities.[13] The problem of misdiagnosis is related to the fact that the symptoms of delirium, dementia, and depression can overlap, and all three syndromes have the ability to coexist.[14] **Table 1** provides a differentiation among delirium, dementia, and depression.

Because failure to both recognize and differentiate delirium leaves the patient untreated, leading to increased morbidity and mortality and prolonged hospital stays, there are compelling social, clinical and financial reasons to improve the differentiation and care of patients with acute delirium.

RISK FACTORS FOR DELIRIUM

Risk factors for delirium may be modifiable (eg, smoking, lack of visible daylight) or nonmodifiable (eg, age); they can be present on admission or develop after admission.[15] **Table 2** presents the risk factors for delirium by level of evidence. Only those risk factors demonstrating high levels of evidence are included, in other words, Level 1 evidence based on systematic review and Level 2 evidence based on prospective cohort study.[15,16]

Van Rompaey and colleagues[16] grouped the risk factors for delirium into four domains (**Fig. 1**). The first two domains contain nonmodifiable predisposing factors. The last two are situational factors, which may be modifiable. These domains are subdivided into patient characteristics and pathology. Based on their findings from a multisite prospective cohort study of over 500 patients who experienced delirium, age, daily smoking (more than 10 cigarettes a day), and alcohol use (more than three drinks per day) were identified as risk factors for delirium in almost all patients. In the domain of chronic illness, the main finding was a preexisting cognitive impairment, usually dementia. Patients with diagnoses related to cardiac or pulmonary conditions

Table 1
Differentiating among dementia, delirium, and depression

Patient Scenario	Situational Features
Scenario 1: A patient with dementia	
A 77-year-old woman was admitted to the medical unit with congestive heart failure. On admission, she is found to be alert, but not oriented to time. She does not understand why she was brought to a hospital. She was found wandering in the hallway at about 8 PM, with a bed sheet wrapped around her shoulders like a shawl and holding a pillow under her left arm. She told the staff who found her that she was looking for the door to let her cat out and petted the pillow. The staff member touched her shoulder and told her she was in the hospital and needed to go to her room. The patient began to yell that she did not like to be touched by strangers and hit the staff member with the pillow. She then began to cry that her cat was injured.	Intellectual impairment Memory disturbance Personality/mood change No clouding of consciousness
Scenario 2: A patient with delirium	
An 82-year-old man, a patient on a surgical unit, had a hip replacement 3 days ago. He has been living alone since his wife died 6 months ago and admits that he has been feeling very sad and unhappy since then. He was alert and oriented on admission and stated that he had cataracts in both eyes. He says he smokes a pack of cigarettes day and has four glasses of wine before he goes to bed each night. On postoperative day 3, he was showing signs of dehydration and an intravenous infusion is started and an arm board is placed on the arm with the intravenous. He reported that he cannot sleep well on the noisy surgical unit. He is moved to a private room, and the shades are drawn in hopes that he can sleep. On hourly rounds he is sitting at the side of his bed reading. The staff close the door and do not disturb him. On the next set of rounds, the nursing staff finds him incontinent of urine and walking around the room, pulling at his pajama top. He keeps looking over his shoulder into a corner. When asked what he is looking at, he states that there are bugs in the corner having a party. He seems a bit befuddled and says he does not understand all of this.	Rapid onset Clouded consciousness (bewildered) Inability to shift attention Visual impairment Isolation Lack of visible daylight Smoking Excessive alcohol Possible depression Length of stay Possible electrolyte abnormalities due to dehydration
Scenario 3: A patient with depression	
A 67-year-old man is admitted to the surgical unit for abdominal pain and vomiting. During the admission interview he admits that the has not been eating well lately, is tired all of the time, and does not feel like doing anything except to watch television. He used to build birdhouses as a hobby but has not built one in several months. He has been complaining of the abdominal pain along with leg cramps and headache for a few weeks, and nothing seems to help. He indicates that the has not felt happy for about 6 weeks.	Gradual onset Fatigue and decreased energy Loss of interest in activities or hobbies Appetite loss Persistent aches or pains, headaches, cramps, or digestive problems that do not ease even with treatment Persistent sad, anxious, or "empty" feeling

Table 2	
Risk factors for delirium by level of evidence	
Level I Evidence	**Level II Evidence**
Based on systematic reviews	Based on Prospective Cohort Studies
Preexisting cognitive impairment, such as	Age 70 years or greater
Dementia	Previous history of delirium
Depression	Alcohol abuse
Abnormal serum sodium	Preoperative use of narcotic analgesics
Visual impairment	Admission to neurosurgery
Use of an indwelling catheter	Exposure to benzodiazepine
Use of physical restraints	Mechanical ventilation
Severe illness, eg, septicemia	Lack of visible daylight
Male gender	No visitors
	Day of hospitalization
	Day 2–5 for older patients having hip surgery
	Day 9 for all older hospitalized patients

Data from Clinical Practice Guidelines for the Management of Delirium in Older People. Developed by the Clinical Epidemiology and Health Service Evaluation Unit, Melbourne Health in collaboration with the Delirium Clinical Guidelines Expert Working Group. Commissioned on behalf of the Australian Health Ministers' Advisory Council (AHMAC), by the AHMAC Health Care of Older Australians Standing Committee (HCOASC). Published 2006. Available at: http://www.health. vic.gov.au/acuteagedcare/delirium-cpg.pdf; and Van Rompaey B, Elsevier MM, Schuurmans MJ, et al. Risk factors for delirium in intensive care patients: a prospective cohort study. Crit Care 2009;13(3):1–12.

seemed to be more prone to delirium in this study. The domain of acute illness is more complex, with fever (temperature over 38.5°C/101.5° F) and the use of drains, tubes, catheters, and intravenous infusions prevalent in those who developed delirium. Administration of psychoactive medication before the onset of delirium (including morphine and benzodiazepines) was also identified, although three or more medications used in combination can contribute to the development of delirium. Interestingly, they that found a Therapeutic Intervention Scoring System-28 using a cut-off value of 30 indicated a nursing time workload of 318 minutes during each nursing shift (5.3 hours of direct contact) for those patients with delirium. Environmental risk factors were found to be related to lack of visible daylight, no view of a clock, and use of physical restraints. An abrupt change in environment such as an emergent transfer from a floor to an intensive care unit (ICU) was also found to be a factor in development of delirium.

Based on their findings, the research group posited that the ingestion of more than three units of alcohol each day, a predisposing cognitive impairment, more than three intravenous infusions, an admission to a medical service, an endotracheal tube or tracheostomy, no visible daylight, isolation, having no visitors, and administration of multiple medications in combination (polypharmacy) were the primary precipitating factors to the development of delirium. Preexisting dementia has also been demonstrated to increase the incidence of delirium five-fold.[17]

TYPES OF DELIRIUM

Delirium can be categorized into subtypes according to psychomotor behavior. There are three subtypes of delirium: hyperactive, hypoactive, and mixed. The patient with

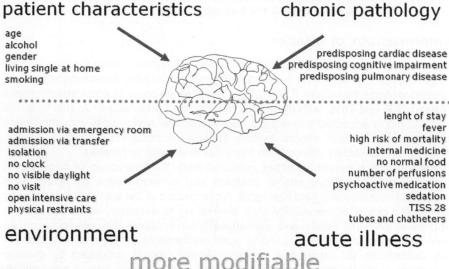

Fig. 1. Domains of delirium. TISS 28, Therapeutic Intervention Scoring System-28. (*From* Van Rompaey B, Elsevier MM, Schuurmans MJ, et al. Risk factors for delirium in intensive care patients: a prospective cohort study. Crit Care 2009;13(3):1–12.)

hyperactive delirium will exhibit manifestations such as agitation and restlessness.[18,19] Frequently, these patients will be combative and uncooperative and may seem to be responding to internal stimuli (hallucinations). These patients will pull at tubes, catheters, and intravenous lines. Hyperactive delirium is seen in 5% to 22% of patients diagnosed with delirium, whereas hypoactive and mixed make up the majority of ICU patients diagnosed with delirium.[20] Whereas it is easy to notice a restless patient who begins to pull at catheters and tubes, it is less easy to notice the patient who is quiet, experiencing hypoactive delirium. Hypoactive delirium is therefore easy to miss and may go undiagnosed. A patient waking from sedation following a surgical procedure may seem to be calm and peaceful but may actually be experiencing hypoactive delirium.[21] Closer examination of these patients may reveal the characteristic inattention and lack of environmental awareness exhibited by these patients. Patients with hypoactive delirium will also present with apathy and lethargy, a flat affect, decreased responsiveness and movement, and/or withdrawal.[22] Often they will nap continuously during the day and do not ask for any assistance. Hypoactive delirium may be misdiagnosed as depression.

Delirium is of mixed type when the patient fluctuates between hyper- and hypoactive characteristics, exhibiting manifestations of both concurrently or characteristics of one type followed by characteristics of the other. The patient may be calm and serene at one point and agitated and restless a short time later. Additionally, some patients may have delirium features without manifesting the complete syndrome of delirium. For example, when using the Confusion Assessment Method for the ICU, the patient is unable to correctly squeeze the nurse's hand when testing for inattentiveness, or the patient has a mental status change from baseline but none of the other manifestations of delirium.[23] Peterson and colleagues[24] examined delirium subtypes in a cohort of ventilated and nonventilated medical ICU patients and found that purely hyperactive delirium was rare (1.6%). In contrast, 43.5% of patients had purely hypoactive delirium, and 54.1% had mixed delirium.

PATHOPHYSIOLOGY OF DELIRIUM

The pathophysiology of delirium is not completely understood, although it seems that the development of delirium is multifactorial in nature involving a predisposed patient exposed to triggering factors.[25] Mortality of hospitalized patients with delirium ranges between 22% and 76%, with the elderly more prone to mortality.[25] At this time, the most commonly accepted premise is a neurotransmitter abnormality with cholinergic deficiency[17,22,26,27] that affects multiple spheres of the central nervous system, although an undetected diffuse brain injury has also been implicated.[27]

Acetylcholine, a neurotransmitter produced from the interaction of choline with acetyl coenzyme A (CoA) affects attention and consciousness by acting as a modulator in sensory and cognitive input. A dysfunction in the acetylcholine pathway can result in acetylcholine activity, thus diminishing its excitatory effect, resulting in hypoactive delirium. Hseih and colleagues[26] have called this phenomenon an impaired acetylcholine synthesis and synaptic mechanisms, where choline and acetyl CoA deficiencies fall under this category. Acetyl CoA is produced by glucose breakdown during the citric acid cycle; therefore, hypoglycemia, severe malnutrition, and niacin and thiamine deficiency can lead to cholinergic deficits. Impaired synaptic mechanisms include nicotine and muscarinic receptor inhibition related to anesthetic agents, anticholinergic medications, and anticholinergic toxins. On the other hand, the monamines dopamine and norepinephrine modulate inhibitor effects in the central nervous system. Dysfunction resulting in excesses in these neurotransmitters can result in hyperactive delirium. Because there is insufficient evidence to refute the cholinergic deficiency theory, current research about the pathophysiologic mechanisms of delirium focuses on gaining a better understanding of how delirium relates to other factors such as hypoxia, inflammation, chronic stress, and decreased cerebral metabolism.[26] This phenomenon may be influenced by the administration of drugs with potent central anticholinergic effects, such as tricyclic antidepressants and antihistamines. Volatile anesthetics such as sevoflurane and intravenous anesthetics such as propofol also have anticholinergic effects and may be responsible not only for postoperative delirium but also for the more complex phenomena of postoperative cognitive dysfunction.[27]

If delirium were solely due to acute medication effects, the delirium would probably resolve after the exposure has ended. However, a significant percentage of individuals developing delirium continue to have symptoms post discharge and are more likely to develop dementia than patients without delirium. This likelihood raises the possibility of an occult diffuse brain injury resulting from local hypoxia, hypoperfusion, cytokine-mediated inflammation, and microvascular thrombosis characteristic of brain organ dysfunction. Certain markers that could be used to evaluate the influence of these mechanisms in individual patients include certain brain proteins (S-100β, NSE, and MPB), and magnetic resonance imaging–detected tissue sodium concentration.[27]

ASSESSMENT OF DELIRIUM

Although there are a number of delirium assessment tools available for use that have acceptable levels of validity and reliability (**Table 3**), health care professionals often

| Table 3 | | | |
| Delirium assessment tools | | | |
Test	Description	Scoring	Population
Cognitive Test for Delirium (CTD)			22 ICU patients on mechanical ventilation
Confusion Assessment Method-ICU (CAM-ICU)	The CAM-ICU is a reliable tool that can be used by nonpsychiatric personnel to detect delirium. It consists of four yes/no questions for use with nonspeaking, mechanically ventilated patients. The exam takes approximately 60 to 90 seconds to administer, is easy to use, and has acceptable sensitivity and specificity.	Four questions	38 ICU patients; 58% on mechanical ventilation
The Neelon and Champagne (NEECHAM) Confusion Scale[29,30]	The NEECHAM Confusion Scale has 9 items divided into 3 subscales: information processing (attention, processing commands, orientation), behavior (appearance, motor and verbal behavior), and physiological condition (vital signs, oxygen saturation, urinary continence). The total possible score is 30, indicating normal function. A score of 0–19 signifies moderate to severe confusion and/or delirium, 20–24 signifies mild to early confusion and/or delirium, 25–26 signifies not confused but at high risk of confusion and/or delirium, and 27–30 signifies normal cognitive functioning.	Three subscales	105 ICU patients; mechanical ventilation rates NR
Intensive Care Delirium Scoring Checklist (ICU-DSC)	This eight-item scale is used for evaluation of disorientation, hallucination, delusion or psychosis, psychomotor agitation or retardation, inappropriate speech or mood, sleep-wake cycle disturbance, and fluctuation of the above symptoms. Each respective item is scored as absent or present (0 or 1) and summed. The scale is completed based on information collected from the 8-hour shift or from the previous 24 hours. A score of 4 or greater indicates delirium, whereas 0 indicates no delirium.	Eight questions	93 ICU patients; mechanical ventilation rates NR

Abbreviation: NR, not reported.

Assessment	Validity	Reliability	Source Study
Table 3 *(continued)*			
44 assessments	Sensitivity = 100% Specificity = 95%	$r = 0.87$ ($P \leq .001$)	Hart et al[28]
238 paired assessments (study nurses)	Sensitivity = 95%–100% Specificity = 89%–93%		Ely et al[1]
253 daily assessments by nurse and researcher	Sensitivity = 97.2% Specificity = 82.8%	$r = .60$ (P NR)	Immers et al[31]
Total number NR	Sensitivity = 99% Specificity = 64%	$r = .94$ (P NR)	Bergeron et al[a32]

fail to recognize it.[18,33,34] The importance of recognizing delirium early in the course of hospitalization is underscored in Kiely and colleagues'[35] finding that if delirium resolves slowly or not at all there is a less than 50% return to preillness functioning. Steis and Fick[18] found in a systematic review that although nurses use several types of assessments to determine delirium, there is a 26% to 83% variance in reporting delirium, meaning that nurses may be able to define delirium but not recognize it in their patients. The investigators concluded that in the studies reviewed (N = 10), nurses are missing key symptoms of delirium and seem to be doing superficial mental status assessments. Silva and colleagues[36] in a study of 111 patients primarily on medical units found that although nurses documented signs of delirium, they were unable to recognize that these signs were related to acute delirium. Consequently, when nursing interventions were applied, they may have exacerbated the condition (eg, application of immobilizing devices). A case study set in an ICU comparing the results of nurse interview, chart audits, and patient observations yielded 50% nurse recognition rate of delirium.[37] As well, Milisen and colleagues[38] reported nurse recognition of delirium after patient hip surgery with rates ranging from 87.5% on the first postoperative day to 50% on the12th postoperative day, which may begin to suggest that nurses are not differentiating delirium over time as familiarity with the patient's responses and cognitive state increases.

Physicians have been found to be equally deficient in delirium assessment. Armstrong and colleagues[29] reported that physicians were likely to conduct only one bedside evaluation for delirium during an entire course of hospitalization. Because of the fluctuating nature of the condition, this cursory evaluation is ineffectual. As well, despite the Society of Critical Care Medicine's promotion of daily delirium assessment, only 40% of physicians reported conducting routine monitoring, with some (28%) reporting that they used the Glasgow Coma Scale or a sedation scale (16%) rather than a validated delirium assessment tool.[6]

Assessment for delirium should occur both initially and ongoing. Because older patients are particularly prone to development of delirium, an initial baseline assessment should be established upon admission. In addition to the usual data collected during admission based on the admitting diagnosis and condition, baseline data should show attention to factors that may indicate the potential for development of delirium including

- Past medical history and the presence of dementia or depression, or a previous occurrence of delirium or confusion, particularly during hospitalization
- Medication history for identification of polypharmacy or the administration of psychotropic medications
- Level of orientation upon admission and any recent changes in orientation or mental status prior to admission
- Presence of any risk factors for delirium.

Devlin and colleagues[30] have suggested that there are a number of potential barriers to routine bedside assessment and evaluation of delirium including the fact the delirium assessments have not been shown to improve outcomes. They also suggest that this phenomenon may be due to

- Lack of clarity as to what health care professional should be doing daily evaluations
- Complexity and ambiguity of some assessment tools
- Lack of clear understanding as to which patients should be assessed
- Time constraints

> **Box 1**
> **Educational Web sites for delirium education**
>
> http://icudelirium.org
>
> http://www.exciteddelirium.org/
>
> http://americandeliriumsociety.org/
>
> http://cra.curtin.edu.au/local/docs/delirium_training_package/ManagementOfConfusionFinal
> March09/introduction.html

- Lack of knowledge regarding delirium presentation and sequelae
- Lack of confidence with using the tool
- Inability to use current assessment tools for heavily sedated patients.

There are a number of strategies that can be implemented to increase the rates of assessment of delirium. First, the team member responsible for daily assessment needs to be established.[30] Nurses are best able to accomplish this assessment because their 24-hour presence at the bedside allows them to detect the fluctuations in mental status, alteration in sleep patterns, and presence of hallucinations more readily than other health professionals.[30,39]

Second, the instrument to be used should be carefully selected. Currently, validated delirium screening instruments differ in the components of delirium they evaluate; in their ability to ascertain the presence of delirium, particularly the hypoactive type; and in their ability to be used in patients with impaired vision and hearing and in those who are intubated and mechanically ventilated.[1,28,34] For example, the Confusion Assessment Method is a widely used and validated tool that can be completed in about 5 minutes but does need training before it can be used effectively.[1] The Intensive Care Delirium Screening Checklist is another validated tool, but it assesses patients for the presence of delirium during the previous shift rather than in real time.[32] The NEECHAM (Neelon and Champagne Confusion Scale) tool assesses processing, behavior, psychological status, and physiologic status.[31]

Educational strategies including the presentation of delirium assessment results during bedside rounds[30] should be considered. Successful educational programs have used social marketing campaigns with resultant increases in knowledge, comfort with use of the tool, and acceptance of the results of the delirium assessment.[2,40] Any strategies selected should include the nursing staff as well as house staff. Strategies used include placing posters in highly used areas on nursing unit, implementation of a kick-off event, medical and nursing grand rounds, broadcast e-mail, and engagement of unit champions. **Box 1** presents some educational Web sites for practitioner review.

Fick and colleagues[41] conducted a feasibility study using a computerized decision support system to improve nurse assessment and detection of delirium superimposed on dementia. The study enrolled 15 individuals with dementia (mean age = 83, mean admission Mini-Mental State Examination score = 14.8) and their caregivers. Participants were followed daily throughout their hospitalization. Results indicated 100% adherence by nursing staff on the delirium assessment decision support screens and 75% adherence on the management screens. These successful efforts encourage the use of information technology in assessing and managing delirium in the elderly.

The most important aspect of a program to increase rates of compliance with daily delirium assessment is the development of a continuous quality monitoring protocol. Indicators related to completion rates, documentation rates, and reporting of changes from baseline should be developed. In general, delirium documentation should be done at least once per nursing shift, and any observed changes should be reported. Quality audits should look for variability within and between providers, units, and time of day. These data can guide further bedside observation and focused education where needed.

Lastly, Devlin and colleagues[30] remind us that delirium assessment and its tools are useful only for screening and that a psychiatric evaluation is valuable, particularly in those instances where the patient's past medical history is unknown or symptoms are atypical.

STRATEGIES FOR PREVENTION AND TREATMENT OF HOSPITAL-ACQUIRED DELIRIUM
Prevention

Successful management of hospital-acquired delirium is best accomplished using a combination of prevention techniques and early treatment with the onset of symptoms. Adequate prevention of delirium lies in the recognition of the risk factors present in the patient, conscious awareness of the numerous potentially life-threatening and non–immediately life-threatening sources of physical and psychological distress that can be present in a patient,[42] and early detection of the onset of signs and symptoms.[43] In other words, a solid grasp of these three aspects of delirium—predisposing factors, precipitating factors, and screening, respectively—will allow successful interventions and quality improvements, particularly because practice gaps have been found in those three areas.[44] This practice can result in improved patient quality of life, decreased length of stay, and lower long-term costs at both hospitals and nursing homes.[45]

Prevention of delirium via prophylactic pharmacologic management has not been shown to be effective.[46] A prospective study on patients admitted for hip fractures due to low-energy trauma found that the use of prophylactic haloperidol in patients at high risk for delirium, based on the Risk Model for Delirium screening tool, was not effective in reducing the incidence of delirium.[47] A systematic review on interventions for the prevention of delirium concurred with this finding[46]; however, it also found that the use of low dose haloperidol does help reduce the severity and duration of delirium, as well as the length of hospital stay,[46] but this conclusion is based on studies in hip surgery patients only. Nevertheless, pharmacologic management may be beneficial, perhaps not as a first line approach, but instead at the discretion of the health care providor when the unique clinical conditions of the patient warrant its use.

Nonpharmacologic interventions have also been studied and seem to be more effective in preventing hospital-acquired delirium.[46–48] A systematic review found that proactive geriatric consultation within 24 hours of hip surgery reduces the incidence and severity of delirium.[46] Reorientation and validation therapy are two additional recommended preventative interventions.[47,48] Reorientation therapy involves using environmental and social cues to promote mental activity in the patient, which in turn helps reduce the likelihood of confusion, disorientation, and therefore delirium. This approach includes using visual as well as verbal reminders of the time, clearly identifying oneself as well as the patient by name during daily assessments, and encouraging and facilitating regular family visits. These strategies have been shown to be successful in preventing delirium.[49] Validation therapy consists of acknowledging the patients' experiences as significant for them, without necessarily agreeing that the content of the patient's confusion is real.[50]

The appropriate sequence of these two approaches has not been validated. Nonetheless, it seems logical that reorientation therapy should be attempted first, because it attempts to address the core cognitive dysfunctions of delirium (ie, acute disorientation to person, place, and time). On the other hand, validation therapy may be needed as the first step if the patient is too agitated or aggressive to allow any attempts at reorientation. If a proactive geriatric consultation, reorientation, and validation therapy do not seem to be successful in preventing the onset of delirium, the use of pharmacologic methods may be warranted. Physical restraints should be used only if there is an immediate danger that the patient will cause bodily harm to himself or herself or to the health care staff.

Treatment

Delayed treatment has been found to increase mortality in ICU patients with delirium.[51] Thus, there is a strong impetus for timely management of delirium. Nevertheless, pharmacologic interventions must not take precedence over thorough evaluation of the patient and surroundings in order to identify potentially life-threatening causes of delirium. Assessing the patient for acute disorders that can cause significant pain is good first step. For example, verifying the position of the endotracheal tube in intubated patients and assessing for evidence of tension pneumothorax, as well as assessing the temperature curve for new onset fever, are all essential variables to consider in an agitated patient with delirium. Checking for non–immediately life-threatening conditions, such as adjusting ventilator settings, applying ice chips to mitigate the discomfort of having dry lips, and adjusting the position of the patient in bed, are also good interventions that can decrease agitation in the delirious patient.[42]

Pharmacologic treatment of delirium is well-studied and includes sedatives, analgesics, and neuroleptics. Haloperidol is the drug of choice for symptomatic management of the patient with delirium.[47,52] Patients with contraindications to the use of haloperidol (such as Parkinson disease, prolonged QT syndrome, or a history of seizures) may be treated with other psychotropic medications, primarily atypical antipsychotics.[53] Benzodiazepines should be avoided unless absolutely necessary (such as in a mechanically ventilated patient), because they are associated with an increased occurrence of delirium.[42] Adequate pain control must be achieved using a patient-centered approach that takes into account the pathologic process as well as the patient's experience of pain. Neuroleptic agents are reserved primarily for agitated mechanically ventilated patients in whom adequate ventilation cannot be achieved despite deep sedation.[42] There is limited evidence for the benefits of using pharmacologic interventions for delirium in terminally ill patients, although haloperidol is still the drug of choice in this setting.[54]

Nonpharmacologic treatments have also been recommended. In addition to the strategies discussed as preventative methods such as reorientation and validation therapy, massage therapy[55] and music therapy[56] have all been used with some success in the symptomatic treatment of delirium. The ABCDE bundled strategy is recommended as a way to encourage interdisciplinary collaboration and the implementation of a standardized approach to mitigate the compounding impact of delirium, sedation, and mechanical ventilation and to improve quality of care in ICU patients.[57,58] This strategy consists of awakening (A) and breathing (B) coordination (C)—an essential part of which are the spontaneous awakening and spontaneous breathing trials—delirium monitoring (D), and exercise/early mobility

(E). Other studies confirm the effectiveness of the different components of this bundled strategy in reducing the impact of delirium. For example, a recent randomized controlled trial found that early physical therapy reduces the duration of delirium in ICU patients.[59]

OUTCOMES POST ICU DELIRIUM

Delirium is an acute condition resulting from a combination of risk factors, chronic disease states, and new-onset pathologic conditions that all interact to manifest as the classic presentation of agitation and altered mental status. Resolution of the acute signs and symptoms of delirium does not necessarily predict a return to predelirium functional mental status. Studies have generally measured certain specific outcome variables: length of stay; mortality at 3, 6. or 12 months; institutional residence (often described as an alternative living situation other than home) after discharge. Patients identified as high-risk for delirium tend to have poorer outcomes postdelirium. In particular, these patients tend to have longer hospital stays,[47] higher mortality at 3 to 12 months,[47] and greater likelihood of remaining in an alternate living situation 3 months after discharge.[47]

Cognitive Outcomes

Studies have shown that prolonged duration of delirium is directly associated with worsening long-term cognitive outcomes.[60] In a prospective cohort study of mechanically ventilated patients who experienced hospital-acquired delirium, 70% of patients were found to be impaired, and two-thirds were found to be severely impaired at the 1-year follow-up after discharge from the hospital.[61] Signs of cognitive impairment include difficulties with attention, concentration, visual-spatial construction, verbal and visual memory, and language and executive functioning, as assessed by various clinical tools such as the Mini-Mental Status Exam.[61] Long-term cognitive decline occurred even in non-ICU patients who experienced delirium,[11] and it may be accelerated in patients with prior cognitive disorders.[62] Patients with delirium are more likely to develop long-term cognitive disorders such as dementia than those who do not experience delirium, even in patients without prior cognitive impairments.[63,64] A study on the cognitive consequences of critical illness suggest that delirium may be the precipitating factor that causes patients to cross a threshold that eventually results in long-term cognitive impairment.

Psychological

There is a dearth of studies on the psychological sequelae of delirium after the patient's discharge from the ICU. Nonetheless, expert consensus and case series studies reveal that such patients have an increased likelihood of developing anxiety disorders.[65] Posttraumatic stress disorder, a severe form of anxiety, is often associated with the post-ICU course, but it has not been shown to be specifically related to hospital-acquired delirium. Other psychological sequelae such as sleep disturbance and depression have been correlated to ICU stay but not necessarily to delirium itself.[65] Further research is still needed to determine the extent to which these sequelae are related to delirium.

Quality of Life Outcomes Post ICU Delirium

Delirium is associated with poor quality of life outcomes across almost all variables measured. For example, delirium in surgical ICU patients has been found to be associated with an increased likelihood of having additional complications, as well as being discharged to a place other than home.[66] In turn, institutional residence has also been found to be an independent predictor of mortality,[47] further worsening the prognosis of the patient who experiences hospital-acquired delirium. Some patients experience persistent delirium even after discharge from the ICU and adequate treatment of any underlying medical condition. Older age was found to be strongly associated with persistent delirium.[67] This finding suggests that older patients will likely have poorer quality of life experiences after discharge from the ICU. There is also a direct association between the risk of persistent delirium and the use of opioid and haloperidol during ICU admission.[67] Other morbidities have been associated with the ICU stay but not directly correlated with delirium,[68] such as the psychological sequelae of the ICU experience and the burden on caregivers, various neurocognitive impairments, the impact of depression and anxiety, and psychosocial distress. There is a clear need for further research on the specific impact of delirium post ICU discharge. Delirium needs to be analyzed as an independent variable from the remainder of the ICU experience because it is not supposed to be an expected component of that experience.

SUMMARY

The health care costs for patients with delirium were estimated to be more than double the costs for patients without delirium and potentially exceeded the costs for falls, diabetes mellitus, and hip fractures[69]; yet the fluctuating nature of the condition makes it a difficult condition for health professionals to recognize and treat. The key, then, is in recognition and prevention.

REFERENCES

1. Ely EW. Confusion assessment method for ICU (CAM-ICU) (Revised). Nashville (TN): Vanderbilt University; 2010. Available at: http://www.icudelirium.org. Accessed September 30, 2011.
2. Ely EW, Gautam S, Margolin R, et al. The impact of delirium in the intensive care unit on hospital length of stay. Intensive Care Med 2001;27:1892–1900.
3. US Department of Health and Human Services. 2004 CMS statistics (CMS Publication No 03445). Washington, DC: Centers for Medicare and Medicaid Services; 2004.
4. Adamis D, Martin FC, Treloar A, et al. Capacity, consent, and selection bias in a study of delirium. J Med Ethics 2005;31:137–43.
5. Rothschild JM, Leape LL. The nature and extent of medical injury in older patients: executive summary. Washington, DC: Public Policy Institute, AARP; 2000.
6. Ely EW, Shintani A, Truman B, et al. Delirium as a predictor of mortality in mechanically ventilated patients in the intensive care unit. JAMA 2004;291:1753–62.
7. McAvay GJ, Van Ness PH, Bogardus ST, et al. Older adults discharged from the hospital with delirium: 1-year outcomes. J Am Geriatr Soc 2006;54:1245–50.
8. Milbrandt EB, Deppen S, Harrison PL, et al. Costs associated with delirium in mechanically ventilated patients. Crit Care Med 2004;32:955–62.
9. Namen AM, Ely EW, Tatter SB, et al. Predictors of successful extubation in neurosurgical patients. Am J Respir Crit Care Med 2001;163:658–64.
10. Salam A, Tilluckdharry L, Amoateng-Adjepong Y, et al. Neurologic status, cough, secretions and extubation outcomes. Intensive Care Med 2004;30:1334–9.
11. Jackson JC, Gordon SM, Hart RP, et al. The association between delirium and cognitive decline: a review of the empirical literature. Neuropsychol Rev 2004;14: 87–98.

12. American Psychiatric Association. Diagnostic and statistical manual of mental disorders. 4th edition. Washington (DC): American Psychiatric Association; 1994.
13. World Health Organization. Depression. What is depression? Available at: http://www.who.int/mental_health/management/depression/definition/en/. Accessed September 30, 2011.
14. Samuels SC, Evers MM. Pragmatic guidance for managing a common, confounding and sometimes lethal condition. Geriatrics 2002;57(6):33–44.
15. Clinical Practice Guidelines for the Management of Delirium in Older People. Developed by the Clinical Epidemiology and Health Service Evaluation Unit, Melbourne Health in collaboration with the Delirium Clinical Guidelines Expert Working Group. Commissioned on behalf of the Australian Health Ministers' Advisory Council (AHMAC), by the AHMAC Health Care of Older Australians Standing Committee (HCOASC). Published 2006. Available at: http://www.health.qld.gov.au/cpic/documents/dem_clin_gline_dem.pdf and http://ccforum.com/content/13/3/R77. Accessed September 30, 2011.
16. Van Rompaey B, Elsevier MM, Schuurmans MJ, et al. Risk factors for delirium in intensive care patients: a prospective cohort study. Crit Care 2009;13 (3):1–12. Available at: http://ccforum.com/content/13/3/R77. Accessed September 30, 2011.
17. Elie M, Cole MG, Primeau FJ, et al. Delirium risk factors in elderly hospitalized patients. J Gen Intern Med 1998;13:204–12.
18. Steis MR, Fick DM. Are nurses recognizing delirium? A systematic review. J Gerentol Nurs 2008;34(9):40–8.
19. Top 10 Teaching tips for delirium monitoring. Available at: http://www.mc.vanderbuilt.edu/icudelirium/assessment.html. Last edited by EWEE May 10, 2011. Accessed September 30, 2011.
20. NANDA International. Nursing diagnosis: definitions and classification 2009–2011. Oxford (England): Wiley-Blackwell; 2009.
21. de Rooij1 SE, Schuurmans MJ, van der Mast RC, et al. Clinical subtypes of delirium and their relevance for clinical practice: a systematic review. Int J Geriatr Psychiatry 2005;20:609–15.
22. Meagher DJ, Trzepacz PT. Motoric subtypes of delirium. Semin Clin Neuropsychiatry 2000;5:75–85.
23. Miller C. Nursing for wellness in older adults. 6th edition. Philadelphia: Lippincott Williams & Wilkins; 2012.
24. Peterson JF, Pun BT, Dittus RS, et al. Delirium and its motoric subtypes: a study of 614 critically ill patients. J Am Geriatr Soc 2006;54:479–84.
25. Miller M. Evaluation and management of delirium in hospitalized older patients. Am Fam Physician 2008;78(11):1265–70.
26. Hseih T, Fong, T, Marcantonio, E, et al. Cholinergic deficiency hypothesis in delirium: a synthesis of current evidence. J Gerontol A Biol Sci Med Sci 2008;63(7):764–72.
27. Milbrandt EB, Augus DC. Bench-to-bedside review: critical illness-associated cognitive dysfunction – mechanisms, markers, and emerging therapeutics. Crit Care 2006;10(6):238.
28. Hart RP, Levenson JL, Sessler CN, et al. Validation of a cognitive test for delirium in medical ICU patients. Psychosomatics 1996 37:533–46.
29. Armstrong SC, Cozza KL, Wantanable KS. The misdiagnosis of delirium. Psychosomatics 1997;38:433–9.
30. Devlin J, Fong J, Fraser G, et al. Delirium assessment in the critically ill. Intensive Care Med 2007;33:929–40.

31. Immers HE, Schuurrmans MJ, vande Bijl JJ. Recognition of delirium in ICU patients: a diagnostic study of the NEECHAM confusion scale in ICU patients. BMC Nurs 2005;4:7.

32. Bergeron N, Dubois MJ, Dumont M, et al. Intensive Care Delirium Screening Checklist: evaluation of a new screening tool. Intensive Care Med 2001;27:859–64.

33. Inouye SK, Foreman MD, Mion LC, et al. Nurses' recognition of delirium and its symptoms: comparison of nurse and researcher ratings. Arch Intern Med 2001;161: 2467–73.

34. Rolfson DB, McElhaney JE, Jhangri GS, et al. Delirium: validity of the Confusion Assessment Method in postoperative delirium in the elderly. Int Psychogeriatr 1999; 11:431–8.

35. Kiely DK, Jones RN, Bergerman MA, et al. Association between delirium resolution and functional recovery among newly admitted postacute facility patients. J. Gerontol A Biol Sci Med Sci 2006.;61(2):204–8.

36. Silva RC, Silva AA, Marques PA. Analysis of a health team's records and nurses' perception concerning signs and symptoms of delirium, Rev Lat Am Enfermagem 2011;19(I):819.

37. Eden BM, Foreman MD. Problems associated with underrecognition of delirium in critical care: a case study. Heart Lung 1996;25,388–400.

38. Milisen K, Foreman MD, Wouters B, et al. Documentation of delirium in elderly patients with hip fracture. J Gerontol Nurs 2002;28(11):23–9.

39. Justic M. Does ICU psychosis really exist? Crit Care Nurse 2000;20:28–37.

40. Pun BT, Gordon SM, Peterson JF, et al. Large-scale implementation of sedation and delirium monitoring in the intensive care unit: a report from two medical centers. Crit Care Med 2005;33:1199–205.

41. Fick DM, Steis MR, Mion LC, et al. Computerized decision support for delirium superimposed on dementia in older adults. J Gerontol Nurs 2010;37(4):39–47.

42. Honiden S, Siegel M. Managing the agitated patient in the ICU: sedation, analgesia, and neuromuscular blockade. J Intensive Care Med 2010;25(4):187–204.

43. Segatore M, Adams D. Managing delirium and agitation in elderly hospitalized orthopaedic patients: Part 1–Theoretical aspects. Orthop Nurs 2001;20:44–6.

44. Alagiaskrishnan K, Marrie T, Rolfson D, et al. Gaps in patient care practices to prevent hospital-acquired delirium. Can Fam Physician 2009;55:e41–6.

45. Leslie DL, Zhang Y, Bogardus ST, et al. Consequences of preventing delirium in hospitalized older patients on nursing home costs. J Am Geriatr Soc 2005;53:405–9.

46. Siddiqi N, Stockdale R, Britton AM, et al. Interventions for preventing delirium in hospitalized patients. Cochrane Database Syst Rev 2007;2:CD005563.

47. Vochtelhoo AJ, Moerman S, van der Burg B, et al. Delirium risk screening and haloperidol prophylaxis program in hip fracture patients is a helpful tool in identifying high-risk patients, but does not reduce the incidence of delirium. BMC Geriatr 2011;11:39.

48. Ski C, O'Connell B. Mismanagement of delirium places patients at risk. Aust J Adv Nurs 2006;23:43–6.

49. Inouye SK. Prevention of delirium in hospitalized older patients: risk factors and targeted interventions strategies. Ann Med 2000;32(4):257–63.

50. Fagerberg I, Jonhagen ME. Temporary confusion: a fearful experience. J Psychiatr Ment Health Nurs 2002;9(3):339–46.

51. Heymann A, Radtke F, Schiemann A, et al. Delayed treatment of delirium increases rate in intensive care unit patients. J Int Med Res 2010;38:1584–95.

52. Jacobi J, Fraser GL, Coursin DB, et al. Clinical and practice guidelines for the sustained use of sedatives and analgesics in the critically ill adult. Crit Care Med 2002;30(1):119–41.
53. Gilchrist NA, Asoh I, Greenberg B. Atypical antipsychotics for the treatment of ICU delirium. J Intensive Care Med 2011. [Epub ahead of print].
54. Jackson KC, Lipman AG. Drug therapy for delirium in terminally ill adult patients. Cochrane Database Syst Rev;2:CD004770.
55. Richards KC. Effect of a back massage and relaxation intervention on sleep in critically ill patients. Am J Crit Care 1998;7(4);288–99.
56. Chan L. Effectiveness of a music therapy intervention on relaxation and anxiety for patients receiving ventilator assistance. Heart Lung 1998;27(3):169–76.
57. Boehm L, Dittus RS. Reducing iatrogenic risks: ICU-acquired delirium and weakness–crossing the quality chasm. Chest 2010;138:1224–33.
58. Morandi A, Brummel NE, Ely EW. Sedation, delirium and mechanical ventilation: the "ABDCE" approach. Curr Opin Crit Care 2011;17:43–9.
59. Schweickert WD, Pohlman MC, Pohlman AS, et al. Early physical and occupational therapy in mechanically-ventilated, critically ill patients: a randomized controlled trial. Lancet 2009;373:1873–82.
60. Gunther ML, Jackson JC, Ely EW. The cognitive consequences of critical illness: practical recommendations for screening and assessment. Crit Care Clin 2007;23: 491–506.
61. Girard TD, Jackson CJ, Panharipande PP, et al. Delirium as a long-term predictor of cognitive impairment in survivors of critical illness. Crit Care Med 2010;38(7):1513–20.
62. Fong TG, Jones RN, Mercantonio ER, et al. Delirium accelerates cognitive decline in Alzheimer's disease. Neurology 2009;72(18):1570–5.
63. Rockwood K, Cosway S, Carver D, et al. The risk of dementia and death after delirium. Age Aging 1999;28(6):551–6.
64. Katz IR, Curyto KJ, TenHaye T, et al. Validating the diagnosis of delirium and evaluation its association with deterioration over a one-year period. Am J Geriatr Psychiatry 2001;9(2):148–59.
65. Volk B, Grassi F. Treatment of the post-ICU patient in an outpatient setting. Am Fam Physician 2009;79(6):459–64.
66. Balas MC, Happ MB, Yang W, et al. Outcomes associated with delirium in older patients in surgical ICUs. Chest 2009;135:18–25.
67. Pisani MA, Murphy TE, Araujo KL, et al. Factors associated with persistent delirium following ICU admission in an older medical patient population. J Crit Care 2010;25(3): 540,e1–7.
68. Jackson JC, Mitchell N, Hopkins RO. Cognitive functioning, mental health, and quality of life in ICU survivors: an overview. Crit Care Clin 2009;25:615–28.
69. Leslie DL, Marcantonio ER, Zhang Y, et al. One-year health care costs associated with delirium in the elderly population. Arch Intern Med 2008;168(1):27–32.

The Stigma of a Psychiatric Diagnosis: Prevalence, Implications and Nursing Interventions in Clinical Care Settings

Carole Farley-Toombs, RN, MS, CNS, NEA-BC

KEYWORDS

• Discrimination • Mental illness • Psychiatric disorders
• Stigma

Stigma has long been associated with mental illness and psychiatric disorders.[1–3] A consequence of stigma for persons with mental illness or psychiatric disorders includes discriminatory attitudes toward them that impact their social relationships and their ability to obtain employment or even housing.[4] Underutilization of mental health services and discontinuation of mental health treatment by persons with mental illnesses and psychiatric disorders are largely attributed to stigma, because individuals seek to avoid being labeled as a "mental patient."[5] Psychiatric disorders are also underdiagnosed and undertreated in medical care settings owing to the stigma that causes patients to be reluctant to discuss their psychiatric history and may attribute their symptoms to medical conditions that are more socially acceptable.[6]

Excess morbidity and mortality rates of persons with severe mental disorders are associated with lack of access to quality medical care across a broad range of conditions, including diabetes, cardiac disease, and asthma, as well as to routine preventative services.[7] Persons with a mental illness or substance abuse disorder are more likely to be perceived as difficult patients by their primary providers, who are then less likely to prioritize keeping these patients engaged in care.[8] Not surprisingly, a related finding is that comorbid psychiatric diagnosis is associated with higher patterns of emergency room utilization,[9] and adverse events during admissions to medical and surgical acute and critical care units.[10] Acute and critical care patients with comorbid psychiatric diagnosis, including substance abuse disorders, pose unique challenges for the critical care nurses caring for them. As members of the

Strong Memorial Hospital, 601 Elmwood Avenue, Rochester, NY 14642, USA
E-mail address: Carole_Farleytoombs@urmc.rochester.edu

Crit Care Nurs Clin N Am 24 (2012) 149–156
doi:10.1016/j.ccell.2012.01.009
0899-5885/12/$ – see front matter © 2012 Elsevier Inc. All rights reserved.

health care team, critical care nurses work with patients most intensely over an extended period of time and therefore are in the best position to recognize and respond to symptoms of psychiatric disorders.[11]

The elimination of stigma toward mental illness was prioritized in the Surgeon General's Report on Mental Health in 1999[12] and in the President's New Freedom Commission on Mental Health in 2003[13] as necessary to achieve the goal of assisting persons with mental illness to lead functional and productive lives. However, a review of the literature in psychology, nursing, and medicine reveal very few clinical trials upon which to build a level of evidence to guide stigma-reducing interventions in nursing practice.[2] This paper explores the stigma associated with psychiatric disorders and mental illness as a social phenomenon with implications for the care and treatment of this patient population in acute and critical care medical settings. Strategies for minimizing the effect of stigma to support improved patient outcomes are reviewed and discussed.

UNDERSTANDING STIGMA

Stigma is a complex phenomenon with significant implications for the lives of those who are affected by it. Stigma can be defined as a "label" that links a person with undesirable characteristics based on stereotypes. Link and Phelan[14] propose that stigma is the result of the convergence of several interrelated components: People distinguish and label human differences; dominant cultural beliefs link labeled persons to undesirable characteristics leading to stereotypes; labeled persons are placed in categories that serve to distinguish "them" from "us"; and labeled persons experience status loss and discrimination owing to judgments others make about them that are based on stereotypes, leading to unequal outcomes.[14]

Most human differences that place individuals in different groups within the population are mainly ignored or considered irrelevant because the differences are generally consistent with socially acceptable norms.[14] However, in a stigmatizing process, a group of people identified as sharing common traits are labeled and that label is linked to a set of undesirable characteristics that are inconsistent with socially acceptable cultural norms. Corrigan and associates[15] identified stereotypes that are especially problematic for persons with mental illness as:

1. People with mental illness are dangerous and should be avoided;
2. People with mental illness are to blame for the disabilities that arise from weak character; and
3. People with mental illness are incompetent and require authority figures to make decisions for them.

The Lived Experience of Stigma

Such stereotypes set individuals with the label apart from the general population, and provide a rationale for devaluing them as persons and rejecting and excluding them from normal social contexts.[1] The stigmatized individual is reduced from a whole and fully realized person to a tainted and discounted one.[16] Individuals with mental illness not only have to deal with the difficulties resulting from their symptoms, but also the limits that stigma inflicts on their opportunities to engage productively with others to improve their lives.[1] Results from research focused on the personal experience of being labeled as mentally ill reveal that the majority perceive themselves as stigmatized by others, expect to be treated poorly by others, and suffer demoralization and poor self-images owing internalization of the stigma attributes.[14–16]

Wahl[17] explored personal experiences of discrimination attributed to the stigma of associated with psychiatric disorders. Respondents were solicited through the newsletter of the National Alliance for the Mentally Ill. More than 1300 persons with mental illness from across the United States completed the questionnaires about their experience stigma and discrimination. Almost 80% of the sample reported direct experience with stigma, including overhearing people make offensive comments about mental illness. Seventy percent of the sample reported being treated as less competent by others once their illness was known.

Scambler[18] differentiated between "felt stigma" and "enacted stigma" in his work with patients with epilepsy. Felt stigma, also called internal or self-stigmatization, refers to the expectation of discrimination that prevents people from sharing about their experiences and impedes help-seeking behaviors. Felt stigma contributes to social withdrawal and the restriction of potential sources of support. Enacted stigma, also referred to as external stigma or discrimination, refers to the experience of unfair treatment by others. The unfair treatment includes condescending paternalism, disparagement and blaming, and fear and avoidance. These behaviors pose barriers to the level of trust and communication needed to understand, assess, and respond to the medical needs of patients, particularly in acute and critical care settings, to support positive patient outcomes.

COMORBID PSYCHIATRIC DISORDERS IN ACUTE AND CRITICAL CARE

Approximately 30% of the population in the United States carries a diagnosis of a psychiatric or addictive disorder in a given year.[12] About 19% of the adult population has a mental disorder alone, 6% have both psychiatric and substance abuse disorders, and 6% have a substance abuse disorder only.[12] Persons with psychiatric disorders and substance abuse disorders tend to have poorer health in general, are at risk for intentional and unintentional injury, and have an increased use of emergency room services.[9] The frequency of comorbid psychiatric disorders in intensive care patients (28%) was found to be consistent with the overall population prevalence when patients were identified through previous outpatient visits with a psychiatric diagnosis code.[10] This process of identifying intensive care patients with a comorbid psychiatric disorder yielded a higher and more accurate number than identification through secondary hospital diagnosis.[6] This finding is consistent with the premise that individuals seek to avoid the stigma associated with psychiatric disorders by not disclosing their histories and/or attributing their current symptoms to a medical condition.

ADVERSE PATIENT OUTCOMES

Depression has been associated with a 13% higher adjusted risk of in-hospital mortality.[10] Medical and surgical patients with comorbid schizophrenia have been found to be at greater risk than the general patient population for adverse events such as hospital acquired infections, postoperative respiratory failure, postoperative deep vein thrombosis, and postoperative sepsis with subsequent admissions to intensive care units.[19] Hospitalizations of patients with respiratory failure and sepsis with a comorbid diagnosis of schizophrenia had at least twice the adjusted odds for admission to intensive care units and death.[19]

Healthcare reform initiatives are challenging hospital care providers to prevent in-hospital adverse events that prolong hospitalization, negatively impact a person's health and functional status, and increase the risk of rehospitalization.[20] These findings underscore the importance of understanding the dynamics that may place acutely and critically ill patients with comorbid psychiatric and/or substance abuse disorders at greater risk for in-hospital adverse events, morbidity, and mortality.

WHAT DOES STIGMA HAVE TO DO WITH IT?

The literature supports the premise that the stigma associated with psychiatric disorders contributes to underutilization of mental health services and treatment by those who could benefit from it for fear of being labeled.[1,5] Untreated or undertreated symptoms of mental illness may include anxiety, agitation, cognitive distortions, and social withdrawal. These symptoms become barriers to the communication between patients and their care providers, and impede ongoing assessment and timely responses and interventions. Anticipation by stigmatized individuals of discriminatory attitudes on the part of healthcare providers can contribute to withholding, defensive, demanding, or hostile behaviors that further erode the patient–caregiver relationship, increasing the potential for adverse patient outcomes.

A study conducted by Hahn and co-workers[8] found that primary care providers rated 15% of their patients as difficult. Providers rated 64 (25%) of 252 patients with mental disorders as difficult compared with 32 (8.5%) of 375 patients with no disorder. Multisomatoform disorder, probable alcohol abuse or dependence, and panic disorder were independently associated with difficulty, whereas association with depression approached significance.[(p4)] Providers described feeling ill at ease with difficult patients and often felt manipulated. About one third of those deemed difficult patients were considered self-destructive or difficult to communicate with. Many of the patients identified by their providers as difficult were very dissatisfied with the care they received. Once the pattern of labeling and reaction is set in motion, the behaviors of clinicians and patients toward each other often becomes automatic,[16] affecting communication, the patient–clinician relationship, and patient outcomes.

ISSUES IN CRITICAL CARE SETTINGS

It is important to explore the interaction between patient factors such as aggressive-ness, withdrawal, anxiety, agitation, and family support and clinician factors such as training, experience, and attitudes for this subset general patient population, partic-ularly in acute medical, surgical, and critical care settings.[18] The presence of comorbid psychiatric disorders may affect communication between the patient and clinicians, influencing how information about current symptoms and prior medical conditions is conveyed and understood. Clinicians may mistakenly dismiss symp-toms of an acute medical or surgical condition, attributing the symptoms to the psychiatric illness.[18] Or, somatic complaints may be attributed to medical conditions, leading to more aggressive care than may be indicated.

Moser and colleagues[11] conducted a large study to examine how nurses in critical care units recognized and managed anxiety in their patients. Nurses in the sample most commonly reported using behavioral signs and symptoms to identify anxiety. Behavioral indicators consisted of 3 subcategories: Agitation/tension, failure to cooperate with care, and changes in verbalization. Among the psychological/ emotional indicators, the most commonly reported individual indicator was anger/ hostility (p. 281). The primary intervention reported by the nurses to address anxiety was the administration of anxiolytic/sedative drugs or pain medication.

Although anxiety is a normal part of life and most people experience more intensely during stressful life events, underdiagnosis of anxiety disorders in medical settings is due, at least in part, to the stigma associated with psychiatric disorders.[6] Alcohol and drug abuse disorders are also underdiagnosed and, therefore, not proactively treated during medical admissions. Use of anxiolytic and psychotropic medications to control agitated or aggressive behaviors without a clear understanding of the psychiatric or substance abuse diagnosis being treated may contribute to a higher risk of delirium and other adverse outcomes related to reduced mobility and medication side effects. For patients with comorbid psychotic, major depressive, and bipolar disorders, underdiagnosis of comorbid psychiatric illness in critical care settings can lead to discontinuation of psychotropic medications during admission. This can exacerbate the patient's psychiatric symptoms, negatively impacting the patient's hospital course, including an increased risk for suicide attempts.

THE RECOVERY PARADIGM IN MENTAL HEALTH

Efforts to change the stigma associated with psychiatric disorders and its impact on the life experiences of those affected need to be multifaceted in addressing issues at a systems level and at the individual level.[14] However, an approach to change must begin by changing deeply held attitudes and beliefs that lead to labeling, stereotyping, setting apart, devaluing, and fearing persons who have a psychiatric illness.[13] In 2008, in response to the national call to eliminate the stigma associated with mental illness, the Substance Abuse and Mental Health Administration changed the name of their educational and resource initiative to eliminate stigma from *Resource Center to Address Stigma and Discrimination* to the *Resource Center to Promote Acceptance, Dignity and Social Inclusion Associated with Mental Illness*. This change in name reflects a strategic plan to combat stigma through infusing recovery-oriented principles into the language of mental illness.[21]

Similar to previous successful campaigns to eliminate the stigma associated with a cancer diagnosis through a shift in paradigm from "cancer victim" toward "cancer survivor," a recovery-oriented approach to mental illness promotes a strengths-based vision that recognizes the importance of a caring, welcoming, and supportive environment to promote wellness and recovery for people with mental health illness.[22]

Ridgway[23] describes the recovery paradigm for persons with mental illness as a process that involves a reawakening of hope after despair and a shift toward active participation, engagement, and coping rather than passive adjustment and withdrawal. Applying a recovery paradigm, a person with a psychiatric disorder can reclaim a positive sense of self, moving from alienation from normal social contexts to a sense of meaning and the ability to contribute to society. The term recovery in this context is more complex and less linear than term used in usual medical–surgical language.[24]

Although some people who recover from an acute episode of psychosis or major depression may feel vulnerable to future episodes, similar to persons recovering from a myocardial event, they often return to previous functioning without significant impairment. However, their risk of a future episode may increase If their previous episode is kept a secret and early warning signs of another episode are denied or ignored because of the stigma associated with psychiatric illnesses. Others may experience significant impairment related to mental illness over many years before recovering the ability to function effectively on their own behalf. Hope of recovery and the social support to achieve it are instrumental in improving their health and functional ability.

The recovery paradigm in mental illness seeks to change the social dynamics that contribute to the stigma that impede the people with psychiatric disorders from participating fully as members of the social community. The recovery paradigm aims to eliminate the self-stigma that prevents people from seeking and engaging in mental health treatment due to fear of being labeled as a "psych patient" and its association with hopelessness, dangerousness, and incompetence. It also aims to eliminate the "enacted stigma," which contributes to inequitable distribution of resources from funding for mental health care that affect access to quality care at a systems level to lack of patience and understanding needed on an interpersonal level by healthcare clinicians to support improved patient outcomes.

RESPONDING VERSUS REACTING TO IMPROVE PATIENT OUTCOMES

Symptoms of psychiatric disorders can severely impair the communication between patient and clinician. A diagnosis of a psychotic disorder has the strongest association with dangerousness, invoking reactions of fear and distancing by others, contributing to social isolation and often resulting in limited social supports during episodes of acute medical or surgical care. Symptoms of other psychiatric disorders, such as major depression, bipolar disorder, and personality disorders contribute to high-risk, self-harming, and suicidal behaviors that result in the need for critical care intervention. The stigma associated with self-harming behaviors can challenge the most experienced nurses in their attempt to be compassionately responsive in critical care settings.

A systems approach to assist critical care nurses and providers to provide optimal care to this patient population involves access to Psychiatric Consultation Liaison Services (PCLS). Clinicians on a psychiatric consultation liaison service provide psychiatric evaluations when patients are clinically able to interact and engage in the process. Based on the findings from the evaluation, collateral information from families and treatment providers, and a review of the patient's psychiatric history, PCLS clinicians can provide an accurate diagnosis and make recommendations to the critical care team regarding medication management and other interventions. In addition to direct patient consultation, PCLS Psychiatric Nurse Practitioners or Psychiatric Clinical Nurse Specialists can also provide education and support to the critical care nursing staff and assist with care plans to improve the care experience for nurses and for patients.[25]

Given the lack of attention in the empirical literature to the issue of mental health stigma, the best approaches for reducing the impact of stigma associated with mental disorders on nursing care in critical care settings is unknown.[2] Didactic education contributes to increased awareness, but has not been empirically associated with a decrease in stigmatizing attitudes or behaviors. However, experimental studies suggest that, among the available strategies of policy advocacy, education, and contact with a person with mental illness, the latter may be the most effective in changing attitudes.[1,2]

The efficacy of interpersonal contact in changing attitudes and perception of experiences is congruent with the basic principles regarding the nurse–patient relationship and patient-centered care. Moser and colleagues[11] found that 1 out of 4 critical care nurses used nursing presence as a core component nursing care for anxious patients. The therapeutic use of nursing presence involves engaging and establishing a trusting relationship with the patient through listening to understand and responding. Hagerty and Patusky[26] propose the integration of human relatedness theory, with its emphasis on trust and shared acceptance of differences, into the traditional nurse–patient relationship framework to make it more useful and applicable to the current, fast-paced hospital setting. A state of disconnection results from lack of active involvement with another person contributing to anxiety, distress, and lack of well-being. Connection is a state of human relatedness that occurs with active involvement with another person that increases comfort and a sense of well-being.

SUMMARY

The stigma associated with psychiatric and substance abuse disorders is a formidable barrier to the achievement of health and well-being for persons who carry such a diagnosis or who exhibit symptoms. Attitudes of nurses and treatment providers toward patients with comorbid psychiatric and substance abuse disorders can be influenced by stigma, which can have a negative impact on the therapeutic process and development of trust necessary to support good patient outcomes. Understanding the interrelated components of stigma, including labeling, stereotypes, and discrimination, can help nurses to reduce its impact in clinical care settings to improve the care experience for patients and nurses. Implementing interventions based on the core values of the nurse–patient relationship to enhance understanding, mutual trust, and acceptance of differences can contribute to improved communication and patient assessments in an effort to improve patient outcomes.

REFERENCES

1. Rucsch N, Angermeyer MC, Corrigan PW. Mental illness stigma: concepts, consequences and initiatives to reduce stigma. Eur Psychiatry 2005;20:529–39.
2. Pinto-Folz MD, Logsdon, MC. Reducing stigma related to mental disorders: initiatives, interventions, and recommendations for nursing. Arch Psych Nurs 2009;23:32–40.
3. Corrigan PW, River LP, Lundin RK, et al. Stigmatizing attributions about mental illness. J Commun Psychol 2000;28:91–102.
4. Gray AJ. Stigma in psychiatry. J R Soc Med 2002;95:72–6.
5. Corrigan PW. How stigma interferes with mental health care. Am Psychol 2004;59: 614–25.
6. Staab JP, Datto CJ, Weinrieb RM, et al. Detection and diagnosis of psychiatric disorders in primary medical care settings. Med Clin North Am 2001;85:579–96.
7. Druss BG, von Esenwein SA, Compton MT, et al. A randomized trial of medical care management for community mental health settings: the Primary Care Access, Referral, and Evaluation (PCARE) study. Am J Psychiatry 2010;167:151–9.
8. Hahn SR, Kroenke K, Spitzer RL, et al. The difficult patient: prevalence, psychopathology and functional impairment. J Gen Intern Med 1996;11:1–8.
9. Curran GM, Sullivan G, Williams K, et al. Emergency department use of persons with comorbid psychiatric and substance abuse disorders. Ann Emerg Med 2003;41: 659–67.
10. Abrams TE, Vaughan-Sarrazin M, Rosenthal GE. Preexisting comorbid psychiatric conditions and mortality in nonsurgical intensive care patients. Am J Crit Care 2010;19:241–9.
11. Moser DK, Missok LC, McKinley S, et al. Critical care nursing practice regarding patient anxiety assessment and management. Intens Critic Care Nurs 2003;19: 276–88.
12. U.S. Department of Health and Human Services. Mental health: a report of the surgeon general. 1999. Available at: http://www.surgeongeneral.gov/library/mentalhealth/chapter2/sec2_1.html. Accessed September 28, 2011.
13. President's New Freedom Commission on Mental Health. Achieving the promise: transforming mental health care in America 2003. Available at: http://govinfo.library.unt.edu/mentalhealthcommission/reports/FinalReport. Accessed October 2, 2011.
14. Link BG, Phelan JC. Conceptualizing stigma. Annu Rev Sociol 2001;27:363–85.
15. Corrigan PW, Green A, Lundin R, et al. Familiarity with and social distance from people who have serious mental illness. Psychiatr Serv 2001;52:553–8.

16. Phelan JC, Link BG, Dovidio JF. Stigma and prejudice: one animal or two. Soc Sci Med 2008;67:358–67.
17. Wahl OF. Mental health consumers' experiences of stigma. Schizophrenia Bull 1999;25:467–78.
18. Scambler G. Stigma and disease: changing paradigms. Lancet 1998;352:1054–5.
19. Daumit GL, Pronovost PJ, Anthony CB, et al. Adverse events during medical and surgical hospitalizations for persons with schizophrenia. Arch Gen Psychiatry 2006; 63:267–72.
20. Weinstein MC, Skinner JA. Comparative effectiveness and health care spending-implications for reform. N Engl J Med 2010;362:460–5.
21. Substance Abuse and Mental Health Administration (2008). Resource center to promote acceptance, dignity, and social inclusion associated with mental health. Available at: http://stopstigma.samhsa.gov/archTelPDF/ADS_Brouchure_508.pdf. Accessed November 5, 2011.
22. Corrigan PW. Target-specific stigma change: a strategy for impacting mental illness stigma. Psychiatr Rehab J 2004;13:537–48.
23. Ridgeway P. ReStorying psychiatric disability: learning from first person accounts of recovery. Psych Rehabil J 2001;24:335–43.
24. Davidson L, O'Connell M, Tondora J, et al. The top ten concerns about recovery encountered in mental health transformation. Psych Serv 2006;57:640–5.
25. Yakimo R, Kurlowicz LH, Murray RB. Evaluation of outcomes in psychiatric consultation-liaison nursing practice. Arch Psych Nurs 2004;18:215–27.
26. Hagerty BM, Patusky KL. Reconceptualizing the nurse patient relationship. J Nurs Scholarsh 2003;35:145–50.

Index

Note: Page numbers of article titles are in **boldface** type.

A

Acute delirium, differentiation and care of, **131–147**
Addiction. *See also Substance abuse and dependence.*
  description of, 9
  diagnosis of, 10
  neurobiology of, 118–119
  neurotransmitters in, 119–120
  pathologic cycle of, classes of abused drugs in, 118
    formula for, 118
  tolerance in, defined, 9
Aggression. *See also* Suicide; Workplace violence
  anger behavior and, gradation of, 48
    nursing interventions for, 49
  as concern, 46
  prevention of, anggression-anger-anxiety relationship in, 47
  relationship with anger and anxiety, 47–48
  risk for, health care workers, 46–47
    nurses, 47
Alcohol intoxication, impact on multisystem organ failure, 3
Alcohol use and abuse, complications of, 3
  definition of, 2
  dependence, criteria for, 2
  effect on critically ill burn patients, **1–7**
  in patients with major burns, 4
Alcohol withdrawal syndrome, assessment of, 5
  benzodiazepines for, 5
  in burn patient admitted to critical care uint, 4
    management of, 2, 4
Amnestic disorders, medical disorders and, 59
Anxiety disorders, medical disorders and, 63, 68–70

B

Benzodiazepine withdrawal syndrome, assessment scale for, 21, 23
  for management of, 5
Bipolar disorder I and bipolar disorder II, medical disorders and, 67
Breathing-related sleep disorder, medical disorders and, 73
Brief psychotic disorder, medical disorders and, 165
Burn injury. *See also* Alcohol use and abuse
  alcohol use and, epidemiology of, 1–2
    defined, 1
Burn patients, effect of alcohol use and abuse on, **1–7**

Crit Care Nurs Clin N Am 24 (2012) 157–164
doi:10.1016/S0899-5885(12)00019-6
0899-5885/12/$ – see front matter © 2012 Elsevier Inc. All rights reserved.

ccnursing.theclinics.com

Printed and bound by CPI Group (UK) Ltd, Croydon, CR0 4YY

03/10/2024

01040460-0013